Hip and Knee Arthroplasty

Hip and Knee Arthroplasty

Edited by **Robert Berry**

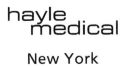

New York

Published by Hayle Medical,
30 West, 37th Street, Suite 612,
New York, NY 10018, USA
www.haylemedical.com

Hip and Knee Arthroplasty
Edited by Robert Berry

International Standard Book Number: 978-1-63241-251-5 (Hardback)

Contents

Preface

This book brings forth an extensive look at the recent advances in the most performed arthroplasties of large joints of lower parts. The remedial choices in degenerative joint ailments have progressed very quickly. Various surgical methods are available, as opposed to yesteryears. Trying to be exhaustive, this book takes up hip arthroplasty with particular accent on advancing minimally invasive surgical procedures. Some difficult subjects have also been discussed. This book would serve as an important source of reference for those interested in the field.

Various studies have approached the subject by analyzing it with a single perspective, but the present book provides diverse methodologies and techniques to address this field. This book contains theories and applications needed for understanding the subject from different perspectives. The aim is to keep the readers informed about the progresses in the field; therefore, the contributions were carefully examined to compile novel researches by specialists from across the globe.

Indeed, the job of the editor is the most crucial and challenging in compiling all chapters into a single book. In the end, I would extend my sincere thanks to the chapter authors for their profound work. I am also thankful for the support provided by my family and colleagues during the compilation of this book.

Editor

Part 1

Hip Arthroplasty

Hip Arthroplasty

N. A. Sandiford[1], U. Alao[1], J. A. Skinner[2] and S. R. Samsani[3]
[1]Specialist Registrar, Kent and Sussex Hospital, Mount Ephraim,
Tunbridge Wells, Kent
[2]Consultant Orthopaedic surgeon Royal National Orthopaedic
Hospital Brockley Hill, Stanmore
[3]Consultant Orthopaedic surgeon, Medway Maritime Hospital,
Windmill Road, Gillingham, Kent
United Kingdom

1. Introduction

1.1 History

Total Hip Arthroplasty (THA) has been hailed the 'The operation of the century.' (1) While the prevalence of coxarthrosis is relatively unchanged from ancient times, attempt at surgical treatment are relatively recent Themistocles Gluck is credited with performing the first hip arthroplasty in Germany in 1891. It was a hemi arthroplasty and he used an ivory femoral head. Early attempts at the turn of the 20th century focused on interpositional arthroplasty using a variety of tissues which included skin, fascia lata, and pig's bladder (1)! Also during this period Dr Ban saw, then chief of orthopaedics at the Mandalay General hospital in Burma, used hand made ivory components for patients with femoral neck fractures. He presented a report of his first 300 cases in 1969. His patients were aged between 24 and 87 years old. Eighty eight per cent returned to sports and bicycle riding within weeks post surgery.

The dawn of the modern era of hip arthroplasty was heralded by the vitallium mould design of Smith-Petersen. Wiles subsequently developed and inserted the first THA in 1938 in the UK.

The next most significant step was made by British surgeon Sir John Charnley. In the 1960's he introduced several pivotal concepts including the low friction arthroplasty, the use of polymethyl methacrylate cement as a grout and the use of high density polyethylene as a bearing surface. While several of Charnley's principles and techniques have evolved, the principles he proposed remain relatively unchallenged.

Arguably the most important modern advancement in arthroplasty surgery has been the establishment of joint registries. These provide invaluable data on survival, complications and can help to establish standards for practice. The Swedish joint registry is the most established of these. Much of the long term survival data for specific types of implants and fixation methods are extracted from this database. Registries are now in existence in most countries including the UK. The American Joint Replacement Registry (AJRR) is currently in the process of being formalised.

2. Indications

The main indication for total hip arthroplasty is pain secondary to primary or secondary osteoarthritis (2), and has remained largely unchanged for the past few decades. Results from the Swedish Registry show the mean age for THR was about 70 years old with a decrease in age seen in men while an increase was noted in women. Recent trends have seen a widening of the indications for performing total hip arthroplasty to include rheumatoid arthritis in cases of failed medical management. Such patients are often younger compared with elderly patients who commonly present with osteoarthritis and trauma (2). Other indications include avascular necrosis, metastatic disease and ankylosing spondylitis.

The use of total hip arthroplasty in treating femoral neck fractures has, and continues to generate controversy. There is a move towards basing the surgical management on patient-related, rather than diagnosis related approach as a reflection of this heterogeneous group of patients. For example, fit elderly patients with pre-existing symptomatic osteoarthritis who sustain a femoral neck fracture should be considered for total hip arthroplasty rather than internal fixation.

There are a number of studies that support this approach. Blomfeldt et al (3) conducted a randomised control trial comparing the outcome of patients with displaced neck of femur fractures, who are relatively fit, active and indecently mobile, treated with internal fixation or total hip arthroplasty. They treated one hundred and two patients with a mean age of eighty years. Forty nine patients where randomised to THR and fifty three underwent internal fixation. Their results showed similar mortality rate of 25% at four year follow-up but a better functional outcome, lower complication and re-operation rate in the total hip arthroplasty group compared to the internal fixation group. Another randomized prospective trial involving two hundred and seven patients by Keating et al (4), treated patients with internal fixation, hemiarthroplasty and total hip arthroplasty. Their results showed better functional outcome in the THA group in comparison to the other groups. Cost analysis also showed a higher rate for the internal fixation group due to higher re-operation rate but no difference between the THR group and hemiarthroplasty group.

3. Patient expectations

The widening indications for surgery have influenced the demographics of patients undergoing total hip arthroplasty and thus, their expectations. More and more young patients are being considered for total hip arthroplasty. These subgroups of patients generally tend to be very active and as result place more demands on the replaced hip. Even the modern day 'elderly' patient has higher expectations in comparison to previous decades as patients are offered surgery far earlier owing to improvement in technology and surgical technique. This emphasis on meeting patient's expectation and optimizing subsequent function has lead to objective scoring systems such as the Oxford Hip Score (OHS), Harris Hip Scores (HHS), the Western Ontario and McMaster University (WOMAC) scoring systems being developed and more recently in the UK patient related outcome measures. A study by Mancuso et al looking at the fulfilment of patient's expectation showed that only 43% patients (of 405) thought their pre-operative expectations where fulfilled fully. They showed that younger patients and those with a BMI of lower that 35kg/m² had a greater proportion of their expectations fulfilled (5).

The modern day THR, however, patient is more likely to be obese compared to previous generations and may develop early failure as a result. However, advances in implant design and tribology have increased the Orthopaedic Surgeon's armamentarium in facing these challenges.

4. Surgical technique

While the ideal approach for THA is as yet undecided, several approaches have been described and are used in routine practice. While no revolutionary changes have been made to the classically described techniques, significant refinements and advances have occurred particularly with the development of minimally invasive approaches for THA and the instruments to facilitate these approaches.

Previous techniques described include the lateral (Hardinge) (6), anterior (Smith-Petersen) (7), posterior (Moore or southern) and medial approaches (8), each with its unique risks and benefits. The approach most commonly used in the UK is the posterior (57%) followed by the anterolateral approach (37%) according to the United Kingdom National Joint Registry (UK NJR) (9). Personal communication with members of the British Hip Society has revealed that the posterior approach is favoured by the majority of specialist hip surgeons.

Results from the Swedish Arthroplasty Register (10) have suggested that the posterior approach is being performed less frequently (52% in 2008 vs 65% in 1992) likely due to an increased incidence of dislocation particularly with the minimally invasive posterior approach. The surgical approach used in our unit is the posterior approach which is described below after a description of the original procedure:

This approach, popularised by Moore, is also called the southern approach. It consists of a 10-15 cm incision centered on the posterior aspect of the greater trochanter. This is deepened through the fascia lata. The gluteus maximus is split along the line of the incision. This along with internal rotation of the hip allows visualisation of the common insertion of the short external rotators on the posterior aspect of the proximal femur. Also visible is a layer of fat which contains the sciatic nerve at its center. This must be protected. Internally rotating the hip moves this nerve out of the operative field.

Once the tendons are identified, stay sutures are placed in the tendons of the piriformis and obturator internus. These are then detached from the femur at their point of attachment. Deep to this layer is the posterior capsule. Once this is incised further internal rotation will lead to dislocation of the hip joint. Repair of the posterior structures is not routinely recommended with this description.

Early criticism of the posterior approach stemmed from several reports of higher dislocation rates in patients treated with this technique (11, 12). Many authors using this contemporary posterior approach have recorded very low dislocation rates and addition of posterior capsular repair has reduced the dislocation rates to <2% (13). Also when compared to the lateral approach, the incidence of postoperative abductor lurch is very low with posterior approach.

5. Dislocation rates

Despite early reports, studies over the last decade have shown that the incidence of dislocation decreases substantially if a posterior capsular repair is performed.

Masonis and Bourne (14) reviewed fourteen studies comprising 13,203 patients. Overall there was a six times increased rate of dislocation in patients treated with a posterior approach when compared to the trans trochanteric , anterolateral and direct lateral approaches. In the group which had a posterior approach dislocation rates among those patients who had a capsular repair was 2.03% compared to 3.95% in the group which had no repair performed. These results were pooled from multiple surgeons however and such heterogeneity has been associated with poor results, particularly among junior surgeons (15).

In a well designed single surgeon series Wilson et al (16) showed that dislocation rates reduced from 3.1% to 0.7% after a posterior repair was performed. Similar results have been reported by other authors (17, 18, 19) including Suh et al who reported that repair of the posterior structures reduced their dislocation rates in revision THA from 10% to 1.9% (13). These results are summarised in Table 1.

Authors	Date	Number in study	Dislocation rates related to approach			
			Posterior	Anterolateral	Posterior with repair	Direct Lateral
Palan et al	2009 (Prospective)	1089	2.3%	2.1%	–	–
Tsai et al	2008 (Retrospective)	204	6.38%	–	0%	–
Kwon et al	2006 (meta analysis)	–	4.46%	0.75	0.49%	0.43%
Wilson et al	2005 (Retrospective)	2213	3.9%	–	0.9%	–
Suh et al	2004 (Prospective)	346	6.4%	–	1%	–
Masonis and Bourne	2002 (Review)	13,203	3.95%	2.18	2.03	0.55

Table 1. Dislocation rates after the posterior approach- Summary of results

6. Our current technique (figures 1-5)

In our unit the posterior approach is used for both primary and revision THA. For primary THA a minimally invasive technique is routinely performed and is described below.

The patient is placed in a lateral decubitus position. The tip of the greater trochanter and the posterior boarder of the proximal femur are identified. A 10 to 12cm incision centered on the posterior one third of the tip of the greater trochanter is made which extends 5cm above and 5cm below this point. The incision proximal to the greater trochanter is angled backwards by 30 to 40 degrees. The incision is deepened to the level of the fascia lata which is also incised. The gluteus maximus is split along the line of the incision revealing the trochanteric bursa which is divided in line with the incision but preserved. Internal rotation of the hip at this stage brings the posterior aspect of the greater trochanter with its attached short external rotators into the operative field. At this stage we use a gauze swab to wipe the bursal tissue and fat off of the short external rotators (SER) attachment gently downward. This action exposes the tendons of short external rotators- from proximal to distal piriformis, superior gemellus, obturator internus, inferior gemellus and quadratus femoris- and moves the sciatic nerve away from the operative field. Next superior border piriformis tendon is identified and a curved retractor is placed under the gluteus minimus but above the superior border of piriformis tendon. Stay sutures are placed in the common tendon of the SER muscles and the underlying capsule (Figure 3). The short external rotators, along with posterior capsule, is then divided with diathermy at its point of attachment to the greater trochanter. Then posterior dislocation of the hip is performed by adduction, flexion and internal rotation of femur. Once the procedure is completed the short external rotators and the capsule is reattached via drill holes to the posterior part of greater trochanter.

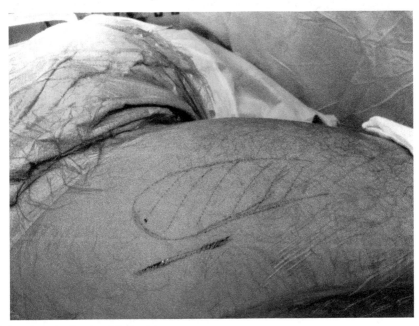

Fig. 1. Landmarks for the skin incision

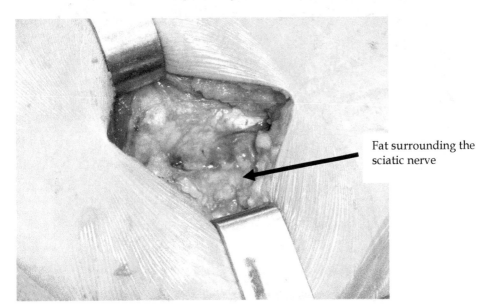

Fat surrounding the sciatic nerve

Fig. 2. Fat and bursa moved away from operative field. This protects the sciatic nerve.

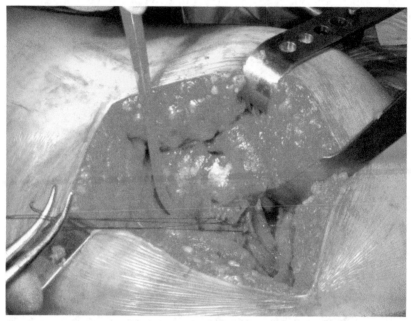

Fig. 3. Stay sutures in the short external rotator (SER) tendons

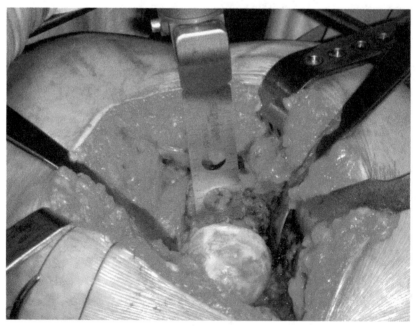

Fig. 4. Dislocated femoral head

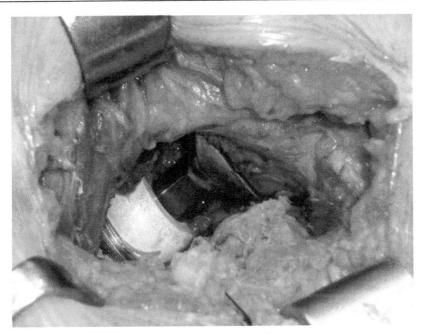

Fig. 5. Post reduction of THA

7. Minimally Invasive Surgical (MIS) approaches

Over the last decade minimally invasive techniques have drawn much attention. These methods represent a refinement rather than a revolution of standard approaches. They have been described for the anterior, posterior and lateral approaches. By definition a minimally invasive approach infers an incision length of ≤ 10cm.

Views and conclusions about MIS THA are conflicting but overall this is accepted as safe, but not better nor a replacement for established surgical approaches. This view is supported by level I evidence. In the UK the National Institute for Health and Clinical Evidence has recommended that the MIS posterior approach is safe but the Swedish Registry suggests that there is an increased incidence of dislocations with this approach which accounts for its decreasing use.

MIS THA has been extensively studied in the literature. Dorr et al (20) showed that while immediate post operative pain control and mobility were improved in the MIS group, there was no difference between this group and those in whom a conventional approach was used at 6 weeks and beyond. Recent level 1evidence (21) has revealed that when comparing the MIS anterolateral, classic posterior and MIS posterior approaches found similar results. This study also found that patients who had the posterior MIS approach had favourable outcomes when compared to the MIS anterolateral approach. Pagnano et al (22) also found that patients receiving the posterior MIS approach walked, achieved independence from assistive devices and returned to activities of daily living before those treated using a 2 incision approach.

While opinions on the clinical benefits of MIS THA seem to be in agreement, these differ on the overall benefits of this approach. Reininga et al (23) in their review, concluded that MIS

THA is a safe procedure although there is no firm evidence of functional benefit. Smith et al (24) reviewed 2849 hips, however, and found a significantly elevated risk of transient lateral femoral cutaneous nerve palsy in the group treated with the MIS technique, again with no functional benefits.

What has not been clarified in this area is the 'ideal' MIS approach, whether specialised instruments help, the group of patients best suited for this procedure and the learning curve for this technique.

8. Technology

A number of advances have been made since Sir John Charnley pioneered the Low Friction Arthroplasty in the 1960s. His design consisted of a stainless steel mono polar femoral stem and a polyethylene acetabular cup both fixed using polymethyl methaacyrlate bone cement. There are currently more than 100 hip stems and cups respectively submitted to the Orthopaedic Data Evaluation Panel (ODEP) for assessment, all of which has variable designs and choices of bearing surfaces.

The National Institute of Clinical Excellence (NICE) which issues guidance on selection of prosthesis advises that the best prosthesis should have a revision rate of 10% or less at ten years, demonstrable by long term viability studies. Cemented prosthesis has the longest viability studies but a number of uncemented prosthesis have passed the ten year mark with good results.

The trend is to use cemented prosthesis in elderly patients with poor bone quality, while uncemented stems are more commonly used in younger more active patients or those with good bone quality in general.

Well fixed cemented components depend primarily on two interfaces; implant cement interface and cement-bone interface. Adequate fixation of both interfaces is crucial to the long term survival of the prosthesis as the load is transmitted via the prosthesis to the cement-bone interface. Any weakness in either may lead to early failure. Considerable advancement has been made from the first generation cementing technique (finger packing, no cement gun, no cement restrictor or canal pressurization) to the third generation (elimination of air bubbles via vacuum preparation, stem centralizer and femoral canal pressurization) thus improving the stability of well fixed cemented implants. In addition, modern day cemented stems are modular, allowing for a range of femoral heads to be fixed for optimal soft tissue balancing and stability.

Uncemented implants coated with hydroxyapatite have either porous coated or grit-blasted surfaces and depend on 'biologic' fixation of bone by bony interdigitation into the stem. A well fixed uncemented stem requires cortical seating into the femoral canal. Some uncemented acetabular implants offer added security of screw fixation for improved stability.

9. Bearing surfaces

An ideal bearing surface has the following characteristics. (25)
1.   low coefficient of friction
2.   resistant to third body damage and wear
3.   generates small amount of particles
4.   has low cellular reaction to wear debris

A variety of significant advancements in bearing surfaces has been made since the dawn of modern era of hip arthroplasty. Figure 6 outlines the major advances.
Bearing surfaces can be split into two broad groups:
1.   Hard on soft bearings
2.   Hard on hard bearings

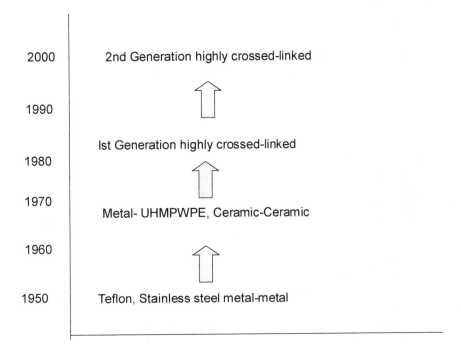

2000	2nd Generation highly crossed-linked
1990	
1980	Ist Generation highly crossed-linked
1970	
	Metal- UHMPWPE, Ceramic-Ceramic
1960	
1950	Teflon, Stainless steel metal-metal

Fig. 6. Major advances in bearing surfaces.

10. Hard on soft bearings

The ultra high molecular weight polyethylene (UHMWPE) acetabular cup was introduced in 1962 coupled with metallic heads to form hard-on-soft bearing surface. UHMWPE consists of several long chains of monomer ethylene which serves to transfer load more effectively to the polymer backbone by strengthening intermolecular interactions. Early wear was a major problem with the early prostheses, particularly with larger bearing surfaces. The third body particle thus generated enters the effective joint space and stimulates a foreign body response resulting in osteolysis which is mainly mediated by macrophages (26). PE wear is related to three main factors; implant geometry and material properties, sterilization and shelf-life. Initially, it was widely accepted that the osteolysis was due to delayed reaction to bone cement (PMMA), this erroneous belief lead to the development of uncemented prosthesis such as the Austin Moore prosthesis. This change did not positively affect the wear profile of the PE cup.
One of the best advances to UHMPE liner use was the advent of highly crossed linked PE liner introduced in 1998. This is achieved by low dose gamma or electron beam radiation

and thermal treatment to increase their oxidation resistance. Its advantages include increasing resistance to abrasive and adhesive wear thereby improving bearing wear rates. Another example of a hard-on-soft surface is ceramic on PE but is not a widely used combination.

11. Hard on hard bearings

Wear-particle related osteolysis around THA components and subsequent failure rates lead to the development of other bearing surfaces such as metal-on-metal articulations. Cobalt-Chrome is the commonest metal alloy used. One of the main theoretical advantages of hard on hard bearing surfaces is reduction in osteolysis (27) by generating less wear particles. In addition, the particle size generated is also smaller (0.015-0.12um) compared to the particle size range (0.2-7um) that has been shown to trigger osteolysis. The first generation metal-on-metal hip arthroplasty showed a low rate of wear and long term results demonstrated that failure was due implant design rather than wear particles (28).

Other advantages of metal on metal surfaces include a higher scratch resistance and larger bearing components which increases the excursion distance, the distance needed to travel before the neck impinges and dislocate, due to the increase in head to neck ratio. This is particularly advantageous in revision surgery for dislocation.

Metal on metal bearings, however, are not completely biologically inert. A number of soft tissue reactions have limited its use. These include metallosis and aseptic lymphocytic vasculitis associated response (ALVAL). There is an increased risk for these adverse tissue reactions in females, smaller femoral head bearings and obesity (29).

Another type of hard on hard surfaces are ceramic bearings, first introduced in the mid 60s. They are harder than metal and have a lower wear rate especially when coupled with its self. In addition, the wear particles generated are biologically inert, eliminating the concerns of sift tissue reactions seen with metal on metal bearings. The main disadvantage, however, is its low resistance to fracture and squeaking, particularly seen in the taller, younger and heavier patients. Like polyethylene bearings, ceramic bearing surfaces have improved since the first generation implants which were more susceptible to fracture.

There are two types of ceramic bearings; alumina and zirconia. Zirconia femoral heads coupled with PE leads to accelerated wear and early failure and is thus not recommend coupling these two components.

12. Results

Total hip arthroplasty remains one of most successful operations in terms of cost effectiveness and symptom relief for patients.

The best prosthesis should have a demonstrable long survivorship and low revision rates. These attributes are best shown by National Joint Registries which not only provide early warning of failures but show cumulative experience of surgeons while eliminating potential bias by the innovator. The main goals of national joint registry is three fold; defining the epidemiology of a particular patient population, providing timely information about outcome and identifying risk factors for poor outcomes (30). The Swedish hip registry was the first national joint registry introduced in 1979. Its main goal was to describe the outcomes of primary hip replacements and to report complications. Since its inception, many other countries have started national joint registries. Many of these registries provide the Orthopaedic community with the results of the oldest and newest prosthesis in the market while keeping track of modifications and innovations.

Charnley's cemented femoral stem has undergone a number of modifications since its inception, including changing from a monoblock to modular stem while retaining the stem geometry. The stem was later modified into the Elite-plus stem (Depuy, Warsaw, Indiana, USA) by undercutting the flange, reducing the diameter and addition of a stem centralizer.

Data for the Swedish hip registry shows favorable results for the original stems; the cohort operated on from 1979 to 1989 had a twenty-one-year survival rate of 81.7% based on 18,607 observations. The more recent cohort, (1990 to 2000), had a ten-year survival rate of 93% based on 20,162 observations (2). Similar results have been reproduced in other centres. Shculte et al showed 90% survivorship of the stem using revision as endpoint in 322 hips (31). The modern day Charnley Elite Plus stem also has favourable medium term results as shown in Kim YH et al prospective study in 194 young hips, with a mean age of 49.1 which demonstrated a 12 years survivorship of 99% using revision surgery as end point (32).

The Exeter femoral stem was introduced around the same time as the Charnley prosthesis and has also undergone a number of modifications since its inception. It is a double tapered, highly polished stem. The Swedish hip register showed a 7 year survival of 98.1% in 4,769 implants. While Carrington et al showed 100% and 90.4% for the femoral and acetabular components, respectively at 17 years using aseptic loosening as an endpoint (33).

Some uncemented femoral prosthesis, such has the Furlong hip replacement (Joint replacement Instrumentation limited, London. United Kingdom) also have favourable results. The Furlong stem is titanium, hydroxyapatite ceramic coated stem first introduced in 1985. Good short to medium term results has been reported in literature (34). The longest follow-up in literature is 21yrs which shows comparable results to previously mentioned cemented stems, 97.4% with revision for any reason as endpoint.

The Corail stem is another uncemented stem with long term results. First introduced in 1986, it is tapered HP coated stem made from titanium alloy. Since inception, it had been modified to a collarless stem and recently (2004) the neck was made slimmer and the taper shortened. The Norwegian Hip Registry shows 97% survivorship at 15 years using revision for any cause as endpoint (35).

These comparable results show that both cemented and uncemented stems can achieve good longevity. Its is likely that these results do not only reflect good implant design but also increased familiarity with use over the past number of years. Analysis of national hip registries show that most of the implants that fail to pass the 10 year mark or with survivorship of less that 90% tend to do so early (2 to 3 years) or at medium term (5-8 years).

13. Current controversies

A review of current orthopaedic literature would reveal many issues of debate and uncertainty. Two issues which currently attract much debate are those of Metal on Metal hip resurfacing (MoM HR) and the subject of thromboprophylaxis after THA. These are discussed below.

13.1 Metal on Metal hip resurfacing (MoM HR)

Resurfacing affected joint surfaces has always intuitively seemed to be correct when contemplating surgery for the arthritic hip joint. The Smith Peterson cup arthroplasty is considered by some the earliest attempt at surface replacement. Charnley in the early 1950's performed surface replacements using thin shells of Teflon. Good function was briefly restored but severe osteolysis occurred in response to high Teflon wear.

The next main thrust came in 70's after THA with conventional stemmed components had been introduced and took the form of metal femoral components with high density polyethylene sockets. Memorable examples were the ICLH developed in UK by Freeman, Wagner contribution from Germany and the THARIES from the USA. Initial results were again spectacular but failure developed because of the large amounts of polyethylene debris.

The poor results of all these attempts led to the concept of resurfacing being abandoned. A British surgeon, Derek Mcminn, aware of how well metal on metal bearing surfaces had performed based on the results of late revision of both McKee Farrar , Stanmore and Ring hips replacements in Birmingham designed a new resurfacing with a metal on metal bearing surface with the metallurgy based on the results that had been learnt from these earlier metal on metal designs.

Contemporary MoM HR was thus pioneered in the UK by McMinn. Improved design, metallurgy and advances in engineering resulted in the design of the Birmingham Hip Resurfacing prosthesis. Original designs have been used in the UK since 1991 and approved by the United States Food and Drug Administration in 2006. Proposed advantages of this prosthesis include improved stability due to its large diameter, improved proprioception, improved range of motion and return to function, bone conservation and relative ease of revision. Early results have been encouraging but data from the UK National Joint Registry (NJR) suggest that MoM HR prostheses have relatively high early failure in certain groups and therefore revision rates. There have been concerns about increases blood levels of cobalt and chromium ions in patients with these prostheses in situ as well as the occurrence of periarticular destructive soft tissue lesions- so called pseudotumors.

Revision of failed MoM HR to stemmed modular MoM THA has also occurred with increasing frequency as a result of the proposed 'ease of revision.' These prostheses pose a new and unique issue to the arthroplasty community as there seems to be concerns with these components which are similar to those for MoM HR. Recent guidance from the British Hip Society (March 2011) has suggested that patients with these components be followed more closely than those with standard THA as the risk of adverse effects seem to be similar to hip resurfacing components. This is currently an area of intense controversy.

13.2 Throboprophylaxis after THA

This is the 2nd area of significant controversy with unique issues in the UK and USA. This issue creates such debate that we have presented a brief review of current evidence before discussing the controversy surrounding it.

13.3 Deep vein thrombosis (DVT) and Pulmonary embolism (PE) after THA

The incidence of radiologically detected DVT after lower limb arthroplasty surgery is 30-60% (for the entire limb) and 10- 20% for proximal segment veins. Symptomatic PE occurs in 1-2% of this group (36). The rate of fatal PE is 0.1-0.2% (37). Risk factors for DVT and PE include obesity, American Society of Anaesthesiologist's grade 3 or above, revision surgery, dementia and renal and cardiovascular disease.

A meta analysis of DVT prophylaxis regimens found that the rate of DVT's increased 2-3 fold if no thromboprophylaxis was used. The lowest rates of proximal DVT's occurred when warfarin and low molecular weight heparin (LMWH) were used. The incidence of symptomatic PE's was decreased by warfarin, pneumatic compression devices (PCD's) and

LMWH. The rate of fatal PE was unaffected. Major bleeding occurred in patients who received low dose heparin (38). This review concluded that warfarin was the best overall single agent.

When used as part of a multimodal approach aspirin has been found to have the same efficacy as warfarin (39). Multimodal approaches address each aspect of Virchow's Triad. It includes the use of regional anaesthesia, PCD's, chemical agents and early patient mobilisation. This approach has reduced the rate of asymptomatic and symptomatic DVT to 5.2% and 0.4% respectively (20). These authors found that patients on warfarin had a significantly increased incidence of wound haematomas compared to those on aspirin. Sharrock et al (40)reviewed >15000 patients and found a higher all cause mortality and increased incidence of non fatal PE's in those receiving contemporary potent anticoagulants (including LMWH, Fondaparinux and Rivaroxiban) and Warfarin than groups who received multimodal therapy.

This evidence seems to suggest that potent anticoagulants are not ideal in patients undergoing THA and conflicts with national guidance in the United Kingdom. It must be emphasized that patients should undergo pre operative assessment prior to a decision on the choice of thromboprophylaxis agent is made.

14. United Kingdom

A House of Commons Select Committee Report 2004- 2005 suggested that 2500 preventable deaths occurred annually as a result of deep venous thrombosis (DVT). It led to the publication of guidance by the National Institute for Health and Clinical Excellence (NICE) on thromboprophylaxis after THA in 2007. Challenges to these guidelines have arisen and include:

- The mortality figures stated in the parliamentary white paper have overestimated the number of deaths
- Using DVT as a surrogate end point for fatal PE has contributed to this inaccuracy
- Members of the guidance committee were linked to the pharmaceutical industry
- Recent evidence has suggested that since the implementation of these guidelines, both the amount and duration of pharmacological prophylaxis has increased along with the incidence of DVTs and their complications (41).

15. United States

In 2004, the American College of Chest Physicians (ACCP) made several recommendations for prevention of DVTs and pulmonary embolism which extended to include the orthopaedic community. The recommendations included aggressive prophylaxis regimens, but were based on the incidence of venographically detected DVTs and used this as a 'surrogate' for fatal pulmonary emboli. In their review process, the ACCP did not consider death and fatal PE as suitable end-points.

Subsequent to the implementation of their guidelines, several centres reported increases in their incidences of major complications, symptomatic DVT, PE, wound problems and re-operation rates, post THA (42).

These reports led to the development of separate guidelines by the American Academy of Orthopaedic Surgeons taskforce in 2006. This group shows prevention of symptomatic PE as opposed to reduction of prevalence of DVT as their end-point. Their guidelines have been considered to be much more relevant, and safer, for orthopaedic patients. This issue is still unresolved in both regions and continues to elicit debate.

16. Conclusion

In summary, total hip arthroplasty is a highly successful procedure in decreasing pain and improving   activity across all age groups, genders and geographic regions. Patient expectations and demands have increase since the advent of the first generation THA but technological advancement is constantly trying to meet this demand. However, there will continue to be controversies regarding the 'ideal' prosthesis, bearing surface and method of fixation. Such controversies may encourage further technical and technological innovations as well as an improved understanding of peri-operative issues such as the optimal method of VTE prophylaxis.
Overall, THA will continue to be a highly successful procedure.

17. References

[1] Learmonth ID, Young C, Rorabeck C. The operation of the century: total hip replacement. Lancet. 2007 Oct 27; 370(9597):1508-19.
[2] Henrik Malchau, Peter Herberts, Thomas Eisler, Göran Garellick and Peter Söderman. The Swedish total hip replacement register. J Bone Joint Surg Am. 2002; 84:2-20.
[3] Blomfeldt R, Törnkvist H, Eriksson K, Söderqvist A, Ponzer S, Tidermark J. A randomised controlled trial comparing bipolar hemiarthroplasty with total hip replacement for displaced intracapsular fractures of the femoral neck in elderly patients. J Bone Joint Surg Br. 2007 Feb; 89(2):160-5.
[4] Keating JF, Grant A, Masson M, Scott NW, Forbes JF. Randomized comparison of reduction and fixation, bipolar hemiarthroplasty, and total hip arthroplasty. Treatment of displaced intracapsular hip fractures in healthy older patients. J Bone Joint Surg Am. 2006 Feb; 88(2):249-60.
[5] Mancuso CA, Jout J, Salvati EA , Sculco TP. Fulfilment of patient's expectation for total hip arthroplasty. J Bone Joint Surg Am. 2009; 91:2073-2078
[6] Hardinge K. The direct lateral approach to the hip. J Bone Joint Surg Br. 1982; 64(1):17-9
[7] SMITH-PETERSEN MN. Approach to and exposure of the hip joint for mold arthroplasty. J Bone Joint Surg Am. 1949 Jan; 31A (1):40-6.
[8] Hoppenfeld S, de Boer P. Surgical Exposures in Orthopaedics: The Anatomical Approach. 3rd Ed. Philadelphia, PA: Lippincott, Williams and Wilkins; 2003.
[9] http://www-new.njrcentre.org.uk/njrcentre/Default.aspx
[10] http://www.jru.orthop.gu.se/
[11] Mallory TH, Lombardi AV Jr, Fada RA, Herrington SM, Eberle RW. Dislocation after total hip arthroplasty using the anterolateral abductor split approach. Clin Orthop Relat Res. 1999 Jan; (358):166-72.
[12] Ritter MA, Harty LD, Keating ME, Faris PM, Meding JB. A clinical comparison of the anterolateral and posterolateral approaches to the hip. Clin Orthop Relat Res. 2001 Apr; (385): 95-9.

[13] Suh KT, Roh HL, Moon KP, Shin JK, Lee JS.Posterior approach with posterior soft tissue repair in revision total hip arthroplasty. J Arthroplasty. 2008 Dec; 23 (8):1197-203. Epub 2008 Mar 4.

[14] Masonis JL, Bourne RB. Surgical approach, abductor function, and total hip arthroplasty dislocation. Clin Orthop Relat Res. 2002 Dec;(405):46-53.

[15] Unwin AJ, Thomas M. Dislocation after hemiarthroplasty of the hip: a comparison of the dislocation rate after posterior and lateral approaches to the hip. Ann R Coll Surg Engl. 1994 Sep;76(5):327-9.

[16] R K Wilson; B Mohan; and D E Beverland. REPAIR OF THE SHORT EXTERNAL ROTATORS FOLLOWING POSTERIOR APPROACH TO TOTAL HIP REPLACEMENT AND ITS EFFECT ON DISLOCATION RATE. Journal of Bone and Joint Surgery - British Volume, Vol 87-B, Issue SUPP_III, 268.

[17] Kwon MS, Kuskowski M, Mulhall KJ, Macaulay W, Brown TE, Saleh KJ.Does surgical approach affect total hip arthroplasty dislocation rates? Clin Orthop Relat Res. 2006 Jun;447:34-8.

[18] Suh KT, Park BG, Choi YJ. A posterior approach to primary total hip arthroplasty with soft tissue repair. Clin Orthop Relat Res. 2004 Jan;(418):162-7.

[19] Van Stralen GM, Struben PJ, van Loon CJ. The incidence of dislocation after primary total hip arthroplasty using posterior approach with posterior soft-tissue repair. Arch Orthop Trauma Surg. 2003 Jun;123(5):219-22. Epub 2003 Apr 9.

[20] Dorr LD, Maheshwari AV, Long WT, Wan Z, Sirianni LE. Early pain relief and function after posterior minimally invasive and conventional total hip arthroplasty. A prospective, randomized, blinded study. J Bone Joint Surg Am. 2007 Jun;89(6):1153-60.

[21] Goosen JH, Kollen BJ, Castelein RM, Kuipers BM, Verheyen CC. Minimally invasive versus classic procedures in total hip arthroplasty: a double-blind randomized controlled trial. Clin Orthop Relat Res. 2011 Jan;469(1):200-8. Epub 2010 Mar 30.

[22] Pagnano MW, Trousdale RT, Meneghini RM, Hanssen AD. Slower recovery after two-incision than mini-posterior-incision total hip arthroplasty. Surgical technique. J Bone Joint Surg Am. 2009 Mar 1;91 Suppl 2 Pt 1:50-73.

[23] Reininga IH, Zijlstra W, Wagenmakers R, Boerboom AL, Huijbers BP, Groothoff JW, Bulstra SK, Stevens M. Minimally invasive and computer-navigated total hip arthroplasty: a qualitative and systematic review of the literature. BMC Musculoskelet Disord. 2010 May 17;11:92.

[24] Smith TO, Blake V, Hing CB. Minimally invasive versus conventional exposure for total hip arthroplasty: a systematic review and meta-analysis of clinical and radiological outcomes. Int Orthop. 2011 Feb;35(2):173-84. Epub 2010 Jun 18.

[25] Minakawa H, Stone MH, Wroblewski BM, et al. Quantification of third-body damage and its effect on UHMWPE wear with different types of femoral head. JBJS Br1998; 80-B: 894-9.

[26] YH Zhu, KY Chiu and WM Tang. Review Article: Polyethylene wear and osteolysis in total hip arthroplasty. Journal of Orthopaedic Surgery. Vol. 9 No. 1, June 200, 91-99.

[27] Michael H. Huo, Javad Parvizi, Nathan F. Gilbert. What's new in hip arthroplasty? J Bone Joint Surg Am. 2006; 88:2100-2113

[28] Schmalzried TP, Peters PC, Maurer BT, Bragdon CR, Harris WH. Long-duration metal-on-metal total hip arthroplasties with low wear of the articulating surfaces. J Arthroplasty 1996; 11:322-31.

[29] Ollivere B, Darrah C, Barker T, Nolan J, Porteous MJ. Early clinical failure of the Birmingham metal-on-metal hip resurfacing is associated with metallosis and soft tissue necrosis. J Bone Joint Surg [Br] 2009; 91-B: 1025-30.

[30] William J. Maloney National Joint Replacement Registries: Has the Time Come? J Bone Joint Surg Am. 2001; 83:1582-1585.

[31] KR Schulte, JJ Callaghan, SS Kelley and RC Johnston. The outcome of Charnley total hip arthroplasty with cement after a minimum twenty-year follow-up. The results of one surgeon. J Bone Joint Surg Am. 1993; 75:961-975.

[32] Kim YH, Kim JS, Yoon SH. Long-term survivorship of the Charnley Elite Plus femoral component in young patients. J Bone Joint Surg [Br] 2007; 89-B: 449-54.

[33] N. C. Carrington, R. J. Sierra, G. A. Gie, M. J. W. Hubble, A. J. Timperley, J. R. Howell. The Exeter Universal cemented femoral component at 15 to 17 years, an update of the first 325 hips. J Bone Joint Surg [Br] 2009; 91-B: 730-7.

[34] Singh S, Trikha SP, Edge AJ. Hydroxyapatite ceramic-coated femoral stems in young patients, a prospective 10 year study. J Bone Joint Surg [Br] 2004; 86-B: 1118-23.

[35] Hallan G, Lie SA, Furnes O, Engesaeter LB, Vollset SE, Havelin LI. Medium- and long-term performance of 11 516 uncemented primary femoral stems from the Norwegian arthroplasty register. J Bone Joint Surg [Br] 2007;89-B:1574-80.

[36] Gillespie W, Murray D, Gregg PJ, Warwick D. Risks and benefits of prophylaxis against venous thromboembolism in orthopaedic surgery. J Bone Joint Surg Br. 2000 May;82(4):475-9.

[37] Murray DW, Britton AR, Bulstrode CJ. Thromboprophylaxis and death after total hip replacement. J Bone Joint Surg Br. 1996 Nov;78(6):863-70.

[38] . Freedman KB, Brookenthal KR, Fitzgerald RH Jr, Williams S, Lonner JH. A meta-analysis of thromboembolic prophylaxis following elective total hip arthroplasty. J Bone Joint Surg Am. 2000 Jul;82-A(7):929-38.

[39] Beksaç B, González Della Valle A, Anderson J, Sharrock NE, Sculco TP, Salvato EA. Symptomatic thromboembolism after one-stage bilateral THA with a multimodal prophylaxis protocol. Clin Orthop Relat Res. 2007 Oct;463:114-9.

[40] Sharrock NE, Gonzalez Della Valle A, Go G, Lyman S, Salvati EA. Potent anticoagulants are associated with a higher all-cause mortality rate after hip and knee arthroplasty. Clin Orthop Relat Res. 2008 Mar;466(3):714-21.

[41] Jameson SS, Bottle A, Malviya A, Muller SD, Reed MR. The impact of national guidelines for the prophylaxis of venous thromboembolism on the complications of arthroplasty of the lower limb. J Bone Joint Surg Br. 2010 Jan;92(1):123-9

[42] Burnett RS, Clohisy JC, Wright RW, McDonald DJ, Shively RA, Givens SA, Barrack RL. Failure of the American College of Chest Physicians-1A protocol for lovenox in clinical outcomes for thromboembolic prophylaxis. J Arthroplasty. 2007 Apr; 22(3):317-24.

2

Why Minimally Invasive Surgery in Hip Arthroplasty?

Antonio Silvestre, Fernando Almeida, Pablo Renovell,
Raúl López, Laura Pino and Luis Puertes
School of Medicine Valencia/Hospital Clínico Valencia
Spain

1. Introduction

Hip replacement surgery is a successful procedure since its commencement. Special attention to minimally invasive access in hip reconstruction has been paid by orthopedic community, implant manufactures, mass media and patients for the last ten years. Nowadays though there is controversy about clinical effectiveness and cost-effectiveness of minimally invasive surgery (MIS) approaches (De Verteuil et al., 2008), many surgeons are using MIS for hip replacement. MIS means tissue sparing, gentle maneuvers, concern about muscles, sheaths, insertions, bone and of course the skin, in a word "preserve tissues". These techniques have supposed an effort for the surgeons to place hip prosthesis with the accuracy of standard reproducible approaches and with a similar rate of complications.

We went through the boom of minimally invasive prosthetic surgery in our Institution seven years ago. Encouraging results obtained by other authors drove us to cadaveric and laboratory training before using this technique in patients.

In the beginning we started with the mini-posterior approach as posterior access to the hip was the most commonly used in our Hospital. We thought benefits for the patients could be obtain from reducing surgical access in terms of accelerated rehabilitation program, analgesic control, blood loss, hospital stay and economic impact, without consequences in long-term results. Good outcomes shown in this paper strengthen our daily work. Four years later in an attempt to reduce posterior dislocation rate after hip prosthesis (around 4.5% in our media and up to 10% in some reports) according to our principle of "preserve tissues", we started using the direct anterior approach with a fracture table (AMIS) in order to perform a muscle sparing procedure that showed a lower posterior dislocation rate than the mini-posterior and standard posterior approaches.

This practice leads us to this restrospective paper that compares our results among these approaches.

2. Material and methods

We evaluated 199 hips (187 patients) which received reconstructive surgery in our Institution. Surgery was performed by three senior surgeons of our Hospital since May 2004 until December 2009. We selected only patients with analogous demographic data and surgeries done by these three senior physicians to homogenize results and implants. No hip fracture was included in this series and diagnosis was primary osteoarthritis in 118 hips and secondary osteoarthritis due to osteonecrosis in 31 hips, rheumatoid arthritis in 26 hips, Perthes disease in 11 hips, mild hip dysplasia in 12 hips and pigmented villonodular synovitis in one hip. The exclusion criteria were severe DDH (different implants are needed) and history of previous surgery on the operated hip that affects functional recovery after hip surgery.

Patients were distributed in three groups according to the surgery performed. Group A included 92 patients (99 hips) who received hip prosthesis through a standard postero-lateral approach. Group B included 46 patients (49 hips) who were operated by a posterior mini invasive access and group C was formed by 49 patients (51 hips) who received a direct anterior approach with the help of a fracture table. Group B and C were performed by the two senior surgeons who got cadaver and laboratory training before clinical use of this technique in patients. Demographic data are shown in table 1.

Implants used in all cases were versafit cup CC and quadra system stem (cementless implants in 73 hips and hybrid hip in 11 hips) [Medacta® International SA; Italy] and bihapro cup and 3-V cementless system stem or PMB cemented system stem (cementless in 98 hips and hybrid in 17 cases) [Biomet; Warsaw, IN]. Bearing surfaces were choose depending on the age of the patients, as we prefer ceramic on ceramic bearing surface for young active patients (under 65 years of age) and metal or ceramic on PE for older people.

	GROUP A	GROUP B	GROUP C
Number of hips	99 (92 patients)	49 (46 patients)	51 (49 patients)
Age	66.19±10.99	66.32±11.72	65.19±13.19
Sex (M/F)	53/39	25/21	29/20
Body Weight (Kg)	81.5±1.7	76±1.9	77.2±1.2
Height (cm)	163.5±2.3	163.4±1.8	162.7±0.7
Body mass index (Kg/m^2)	30.6±1.3	27.8±1.6	29.3±1.1
Preoperative diagnosis			
Osteoarthritis	60	28	32
Osteonecrosis	12	8	11
RA	14	6	4
Perthes	6	3	2
Hip displasia	7	4	1
Pigmented villonodular synovitis			1
Preoperative HSS	57.010 (SD 4.09)	57.959 (SD 6.26)	56.606 (SD 6.16)

Table 1. Demographic data of the patients

Institutional approval was obtained from the Hospital for the new techniques. Learning curve affected results in the beginning of the procedure and fluoroscopy was used during the beginning of these series to aid in implant position and anatomic referencing.

No great changes were adopted for the mini invasive posterior access, as patient position is similar to the conventional posterolateral approach. A more straight oblique and proximal incision was employed for the mini-posterior access. Specific devices designed for the different approaches were used in order to get proper placement of the implants. The cup was inserted in 40-45° abduction angle in the different groups but a bigger anteversion angle was applied to the acetabulum in the posterior approaches to avoid posterior dislocation of the hip. Femoral reaming, broaching and stem implantation were resumed in the mini-posterior access as in conventional postero-lateral approach with the aid of some devices developed to bring up proximal femur into the incision.

Our operative technique for direct anterior approach (AMIS) was the same that described F. Laude (Laude, 2006). Patients were placed in supine position on an orthopaedic table with the foot of the operated leg secured in a traction device (Medacta®). The operation table was positioned in horizontal condition to the floor and the pelvis was checked to be set in neutral angle tilting angle. Towel pads were placed under the buttock to stabilize pelvic movement and to bring up proximal femur into the incision during flexion and adduction of the leg. The cup was inserted in 40-45° inclination angle by referring alignment rod to the interconnecting line of bilateral ASIS and 10° anteversion angle by referring the rod to the operation table. Controls by image intensifier were used during first cases to estimate inclination and anteversion angle. After cup placement, traction and gentle external rotation was applied to the operated leg. The supero-lateral capsule and the pubo-femoral ligament were released for appropriate femoral exposure and preparation. Femoral reaming, broaching and stem implantation were performed after verifying the direction of the femoral axis and anterior bow of the femur.

Full weight bearing was allowed from the second-third postoperative day depending on laboratory results and need of red cell transfusion, except in complicated cases. Walking with a walker or crutches was started from the second day after surgery. Patients were permitted to go up and down the stair using handrail from the fifth day after surgery. Using a cane or a walker was based on patient's ability. Physical theraphists instructed gait training and ambulation during patient's hospital stay. Patients left the hospital when they get sufficient hip function for their activity of daily living.

Operative time (skin incision to skin closure) and intraoperative and postoperative blood loss volume were evaluated as indices of operative invasion. Intraoperative blood loss volume was estimated by using the volume in the suction device adding up the weight of compresses used during surgery. Postoperative blood loss volume was measured by drain output postoperatively, which was removed 48 h after surgery. Laboratory tests were used to determine haemoglobin concentration and haematocrit (HCT) 36-48 h after surgery to get a more real scene of the patient's hemodynamic status.

Standard protocol during the time of this study for all the patients was low molecular-weight heparin for 28 days postoperatively. Elastic stocking was applied to both legs for intraoperative deep venous thrombosis until first outpatient visit. Ultrasound was obtained only in patients with symptoms of deep vein thrombosis. Cefazolin (Kefol®) two grams were given intravenously an hour before surgery, followed by 1 gr/8h for two days after surgery. Analgesic drugs were given during hospital stay but no morphic therapy was used in the immediate postoperatory.

Patients were assessed preoperatively and postoperatively at 6 weeks, 3 months and annually thereafter with clinical evaluation including gait, need for assistance devices, ROM and visual analog pain score. Standard radiographs of the operated hip were taken at 6 weeks, 3 months and at annual review. Radiological assessment was performed by measuring cup inclination, cup anteversion angle and positioning of cup within the safe zone of Lewinnek (Lewinnek et al., 1978). Stem alignment of varus or valgus positioning of less than 3° was considered neutral position on AP X-ray. Hip function was assessed clinically using the Harris Hip Score at 6 weeks, 3 months, and annually. Data are collected pre and postoperatively from patient questionnaires and from an independent senior orthopaedic surgeon (R.L.) assessment at each visit. All known complications were captured and collected for descriptive study.

Differences in laboratory levels, drain output measures, length of hospital stay, visual analog pain score and gait parameters between groups were examined using an unpaired Student's t-test with the aid of SPS-15. The significance level was set at P<.05 for all analysis.

3. Results

Three groups were established depend on the access employed to the hip joint. Underlying diagnosis was ortheoarthritis and osteonecrosis in 74.87% of cases.

Mean operative time was longer in first cases after introduction of the new techniques (mini posterior and AMIS) due to our learning curve, but this rate returns to equivalent operative time value as the standard postero-lateral approach after our fifteen surgeries. Hip access has no significant difference in surgery time [P= 0.44]. The average blood loss during the surgery was 162.4±57.7 ml for group A, 149.4±57.3 ml for group B and 141.5±54.2 ml for group C as meticulous hemostasis was applied in all cases and a sealer device was used in the last group. Measurement of blood loss in drain output shows a significant difference between group C and A [P=0.04] but no between group B and A. The overall risk of red cell transfusion was bigger in group A that in the rest of groups. Average length of the hospital stay that shows significant differences between minimally invasive procedures and standard access of the hip [P=0.023] could be explained by other facts as introduction of accelerate rehabilitation programmes linked to the new techniques. However, absence of skilled nursing or extended-care facilities affects patients discharge to home in our environment. Other indices of operative invasion, hip stability and walking ability are reported in table 2.

Five posterior hip dislocations were observed in group A and two in group B. No hip dislocation has been assessed in group C.

Analyzing hip recovery we checked that time required to single-leg stance for more than 5 seconds was 21.3 days in group A (range 12-76 days), 20.9 (range 10-75 days) and 17.1 days (range 5-75 days) in group C. There were no significant differences in the single-leg stance between anterior and posterior approaches. However this competence depends on patient's age, therapist's cooperation and previous functional status. Positive Trendelenburg's sign was identified in mostly all the patients before surgery, but at six weeks it was recognized in only 3.92 % of hips in group C. Negative Trendelenburg's sign was acquired in this group at 17.3 days (range 5-75 days). There were significant differences between anterior and posterior approaches [P=0.048].

In our series required time up to walking by two canes or a walker was 3.494±1.163 for group A, 2.571±0.912 for group B and 2.262±0.68 for group C. No significant differences have been found among the different approaches. Patients from group C were able to walk by a single cane more than 250 meters at 15.0 days (range 3-35 days) and fifty-six percent of these patients were capable to walk without the use of assistive walking aids at three weeks postoperatively. On the opposite patients from group A and B were able to walk by a single cane more than 250 meters at 19.4 days (range 5-41 days). There were significant differences between posterior and anterior access to the hip [P= 0.039] (table 3).

Harris hip score results are shown in table 2, but no significant differences were observed among the three groups. Visual analog pain score after surgery improved to 3.030±0.984 in group A, 2.489±0.71 in group B and 2.213±0.798 in group C. Significant differences were detected when comparing group C with the others groups [P<0.05] (table 3). Three patients (two in group A and one in group C) developed inguinal pain three months after surgery. An infiltration of the ileopectineus bursa resolved their symptoms.

Ninety-six cups (96.07%) had been implanted within the safe zone of the Lewinnek method in this series (Lewinnek et al., 1978). Less anteversion angle was applied to the cups in the anterior approach to avoid anterior dislocation. On the other hand anteversion angle was bigger in group A and B (posterior access) to prevent from posterior dislocation of the hip. Stem alignment in anteroposterior radiograph was 178.56±0.97 in group A, 179.23±1.13 in group B and 179.85±1.94 in group C with no cases or varus o valgus position (more than 3° in the A-P X-ray).

	GROUP A	GROUP B	GROUP C
Operative time(minutes)	79.25±18.90	84.61±16.47	87.24±30.51
Blood loss (drain ouput)	624.64±10.62 ml	595.91±13.21 ml	579.01±14.91
Need transfusión	22.77%	16.21%	14.75%
Preoperative Hb	13.45±1.32 g/dl	13.58±1.07 g/dl	13.38±1.39 g/dl
Postoperative Hb	8.89±0.69 g/dl	9.3±0.78 g/dl	9.76±1.16 g/dl
Preoperative HTO	39.35±3.64	39.61±3.13	39.06±4.14
Postoperative HTO	26.51±2.14	27.96±2.40	28.38±3.12
Lenght of hospital stay after surgery	7.35±2.04 days (84.8%)	6±1.81 days (83.6%)	4.78±1.23 days (83.6%)
Presence of Trendelenburg's sign			
1 week	87 hips (87.87%)	43 hips (87.75%)	41 hips (80.39%)
3 weeks	44 hips (44.44%)	21 hips (42.85%)	14 hips (27.65%)
6 weeks	13 hips (13.13%)	6 hips (12.24%)	2 hips (3.92%)
Average time to single-leg stance > 5"	21.3 days	20.9 days	17.1 days
No assistive walking aids (3 weeks)	47 hips (47.47%)	24 hips (48.97%)	29 hips (56.82%)
HHS			
6 weeks	72.61±3.23	73.74±3.23	79.27±7.45
3 months	83.82±4.20	84.91±4.96	88.08±6.09
1 year	90.74±6.16	91.15±6.04	91.34±6.07

Table 2. Indices of operative invasion, hip stability and walking ability

Intraoperative and postoperative complications are shown in Table 4. Main surgical complications were observed in our learning curve (15 first cases) of the minimally invasive techniques as we think these are demanding procedures which require experience in hip surgery. Intraoperative complications were detected and settled during surgery. Proximal femoral perforations identified during broaching and reaming the femur in the AMIS procedure (group C) did not alter the procedure. Periprosthetic fractures were fixed with cerclage cable fixation and major throchanteric fractures require cerclage cable fixation in posterior approaches (group A and B) but no fixation was used in the anterior access (group C). A femoral shaft fracture was confirmed during preparation for the insertion of the stem in group C; enlarging of the exposure in zigzag way allowed us to reduce and fixed the fracture with a femoral plate with screws and cables. The case requiring acute revision was cup dislodgment checked with X-ray control that needed re-operation two days after first surgery. Deep infections needed two-stage revision of the hips; the average interval between first-stage resection and reimplantation was 5.2 months. On the other hand superficial wound infections were resolved by superficial debridement and irrigation with wound closure. Lateral femoral cutaneous nerve paresthesias verified in group C improved six months after surgery. The cases of clinically evident deep-vein thrombosis were treated with pharmacologycal therapy. A young patient of group C died two days after surgery due to a fatal embolism. All cases of length leg discrepancy were less than 1 cm and well tolerated by the patients, so we do not include as complications.

	Hb decrease	HTO decrease	Blood loss (drain output)	Lenght of hospital stay	Visual analog score	Walk by a single cane 250 m
Group B-A	P= 0.058	P= 0.2	P> 0.05	P= 0.02	P> 0.05	P> 0.05
Group C-A	P= 0.0001	P= 0.08	P= 0.04	P= 0.02	P=0.02	P= 0.03
Group C-B	P= 0.0001	P= 0.3	P= 0.33	P= 0.007	P= 0.008	P= 0.03

Table 3. Comparative of some results between groups (P values)

	Group A Cases (number) and treatment	Group B Cases (number) and treatment	Group C Cases (number) and treatment
Femoral shaft fracture	0	0	1 Femoral plate (screws and cable fixation)
Periprosthetic fracture	2 Cerclage cable fixation	2 Cerclage cable fixation	1 Cerclage cable fixation
Proximal femoral perforation	0	3 No treatment	2 No treatment
Major throchanteric fracture	3 Cerclage cable fixation	3 Cerclage cable fixation	4 No treatment
Cup dislodgment	0	0	1 Acute revision
Posterior dislocation	5 Closed reduction	2 Closed reduction	0
Deep infection	4 Two-stage revision	2 Two-stage revision	0
Superficial infection	5 Debridement	2 Debridement	2 Debridement
Nonfatal DVT	6 Pharmacologycal therapy	3 Pharmacologycal therapy	2 Pharmacologycal therapy
Stem subsidence	2 Well tolerated	0	1 Well tolerated
Paresthesias of the lateral aspect of the thigh	0	0	4
Fatal embolism. RIP	0	0	1

Table 4. Complications in our series

4. Discussion

Access to hip joint for placing a THA has been gained by different approaches along history. Each one has advantages and disadvantages but nevertheless we can assume total hip replacement is a successful procedure. Different viewpoints and discussions persist nowadays regarding fixation procedures, gliding couples and materials. In this context appeared years ago the concept of "minimally invasive surgery" that must be distinguished from less invasive surgery (Judet, 2006). This background supposed a breeding soil to show immeasurable advantages of these techniques. Plenty of reports were published describing its benefits in terms of economy, accelerated rehabilitation and comfort for the patients. These encouraging results explained the anxiety of the people about this useful surgery. However time has put these procedures in his place (Goosen et al., 2011; Maffiuletti et al., 2009; Nakata et al., 2009; Pospischill et al., 2010; Roy et al., 2010; Sugano et al., 2009). However there are some evidences of benefits reported by minimally invasive procedures (Berend et al., 2009; Duwelius & Dorr, 2008; Khan et al., 2006; Lamontagne et al., 2011; Matziolis et al., 2011; Müller et al., 2011; Nakata et al., 2009; Stehlík et al., 2008; Varela et al., 2010). We believe that with a good selection of the patients and after an education and training schedule these techniques are safe and reproducible.

Muscle damage and blood loss was two our main concerns in hip surgery. We have not established a pre-donation autologous blood protocol at our Institution and economic analysis of this practice was no cost-benefit in our environment. In order to lessen red cell transfusion we start the mini-posterior approach delighted with encouraging reports from other authors (Khan et al., 2006; Mazoochian et al., 2009; Sculco & Boettner, 2006). Though we reduced red cell transfusion with our mini-posterior access (group B) compare to the standard approach (group A) 16.32% vs 22.77% no significant differences were found in blood loss in the drain output, haemoglobin and HTO decrease [P>0.05].

It is believed that muscle protection enables the patient to start the rehabilitation program earlier and to reduce the length of his/her hospital stay (Goosen et al., 2011; Nakata et al., 2009; Palieri et al., 2011; Stehlík et al., 2008; Varela et al.,2010). Our plan was to minimize injure to muscles and/or bone to accelerate rehabilitation but we were not so worried about short scars. We had no doubt in enlarging the incision if it was required during our performances to be confident with the stem or cup position or to avoid damaging soft tissues. After introduction of the mini-posterior approach (group B) decrease in length hospital stay was observed with significant differences to standard access (group A) [P= 0.02], but usually when new techniques are introduced more attention is paid to questions as rehabilitation programmes and shortening hospital stay. We have also found in our series an improving in HHS and visual analog score for the first three months, however without significant differences with the standard approach.

Once the two of our main concerns were improved, we focused our attention in posterior dislocation. The posterior approach, the most commonly used at our Institution and all around the world has a high hip dislocation rate, up to 10 % in some reports (around 4.5% in our media) (Berry et al., 2004; Heithoff et al., 2001; Khan et al., 2006; Peters et al., 2007). In an attempt to prevent dislocations (none in group C in this series), being respectful with soft tissues we looked for news approaches as the AMIS, three and a half years ago. We believe this direct anterior approach, classically known as "Smith-Peterson" but initially described by the German surgeon Carl Hueter, provides an excellent exposure of the hip, is a muscle sparing procedure and has a lower dislocation rate than the posterior approach (Matta et al.,

2005; Siguier et al., 2004). We have no great experience with the antero-lateral approach but even though its dislocation rate is low, we have found more limping after THA in patients with the lateral approach.

As well as lessening the rate of posterior hip dislocations this technique allows a proper exposure of the acetabulum (Mast & Laude 2011) and it is widely accepted. In the current literature few reports have compared the extent and location of muscle damage between posterior and the direct anterior approaches (Nakata et al., 2009; Meneghini et al., 2005). Only Meneghini and colleagues reported a comparative cadaveric study about muscle damage evaluation with both approaches (Meneghini et al., 2005). He concluded that main differences related to injured muscle were in the gluteus minimus, being less harmful the anterior approach (8.5% vs 18%). Another comparative study shows that more patients could walk without assistive devices 3 weeks after surgery with the anterior direct approach (34%) than with the posterior one (Nakata et al., 2009). For that reasons, we started using the AMIS approach that let us get access to the hip through an inter-muscular (sartorius muscle and tensor fascia lata muscle) and inter-nervous (femoral nerve and superior gluteal nerve) portal. The anterior approach, which remains as the standard approach to the hip in paediatric orthopaedic surgery (Berger et al., 2004) regained popularity in adult procedures with the outbreak of the minimally invasive surgeries.

The principal advantage of this portal is that even an extensile exposure was required the gluteal muscles were keep intact. We agree with the idea that "minimally invasive surgery" does not imply short scars but require paying attention to soft tissues (Barton & Kim, 2009; Sculco, 2004; Waldman, 2003; Wojciechowski et al., 2007). Injuries to a muscle or its attachments impair muscle propioception and reduce its strength. Preventing muscle or attachments injure helps restoring normal muscular tension and improve stabilization of the hip joint.

Haemoglobin decreases after anterior minimally invasive procedure shows significant differences comparing this group with the mini posterior and standard approach [P= 0.0001], but no significant results were obtained with HTO. Blood loss in the drain output also reflects significant differences making the comparison to standard approach (group A) [P= 0.04] but not with the mini-posterior access (group B) [P= 0.33]. The reduction in blood loss was attributed to meticulous care with haemostasis to avoid wound hematomas as the only layer was closed was the sheath of the TFL (Morris et al., 2010), however most of the bleeding in hip replacement depends on bone bed not on the size of the wound. It is admitted that wound hematoma formation may be greater in the direct anterior approach as the incision is anterior and there is less inherent pressure on the wound that may aid in hemostasis. We believe that meticulous haemostasis is required to obtain a good view of the joint, so we prefer to use bipolar sealer to avoid bleeding (Morris et al., 2010). These details allow us to control blood loss, give us a neat exposure of the hip joint and let us take anatomic references for accurate component placement.

We found an improvement in HHS (Klausmeier et al., 2010; Lugade et al., 2010; Matziolis et al., 2011) and Trendelenburg's test (Nakata et al., 2009) with the AMIS. Visual analog pain score also improved with significant differences related to group A and B [P= 0.02 and P= 0.008]. Walking ability and length of hospital stay show significant differences comparing results to group A and B [P< 0.05] (Berend et al., 2009; Khan et al., 2006; Lamontagne et al., 2011; Maffiuletti et al., 2009; Morris et al. 2010; Nakata et al., 2009; Seng et al. 2009). Patients in group C were in hospital for a mean 4.78 days with the majority discharged to home (83.6%). Lower blood loss and muscle sparing that allowed the patients an accelerated program of rehabilitation made them more confident after surgery to start walking, sitting or getting out of bed. Our patients used assistive devices as crutches or walkers during their hospital stay.

The concept of tissue sparing surgery has been an important fact in surgical techniques for the last ten years. It includes reduced incisions with small scars, but the real point toward these procedures attempt is preserving soft tissues. These techniques are as much careful as possible with muscles, sheaths, insertions, bone and of course the skin. They suppose new exposure techniques and of course new instruments to place the same prosthesis with the accuracy of the standard approaches and with few complications. Manufactures, tribologists and engineers have done a great effort to make possible these techniques but some of the advantages found in the current paper in terms of patient comfort, anaesthetic parameters, related costs, length of hospital stay, analgesic use, blood loss and patient rehabilitation explain the enthusiasm of orthopaedic surgeons in these procedures. According to the classification of Duncan in 2006, based on approach to the skin, number of skin incisions and technique of dissection the anterior direct approach is an "intermuscular approach" meanwhile the lateral and posterior approaches, with a standard or mini-incision, are classified as "transmuscular approaches" as they include and invasive operating step with muscle and tendon sectioning. Only the double access can be considered as a tissue sparing surgery but sometimes requires new design for the implants and prolonged used of an x-ray C-arm to check component placement. Besides these facts, cadaveric studies suggest greater muscle damage occurs with the two-incision technique than with the direct anterior approach (Mardones et al., 2005; Meneghini et al., 2005).

Zati (Zati et al., 1997) and He (He et al., 1988) concluded that, in early post-operative time, the afferent nerves to the muscle are more important than hip capsule receptors. Accepting that hypothesis tendon sectioning should be avoid because this gesture can affect sensomotory capacity of the joint so rehabilitation programme will be longer and worse functional scores will be obtain. This could explain better early functional outcome scores and visual analog score pain in the anterior direct approach compared to posterior procedures.

Every time a new procedure is established, great concern about possible complications arises in surgeons' mind. Minimally invasive approaches are related to longer surgery time and recommended in selected patients (Vail & Callaghan, 2007). However, a learning curve is necessary to take a new surgical access into practice. We have checked longer operating time in group B and C particularly in our first cases, but not significant differences were found [P= 0.44].

D'Arrigo (D'Arrigo et al., 2009) reported the rate of complications is not reduced along a geometric pattern during the learning curve of the anterior minimally invasive surgery, whereas surgical time was significantly correlated with this learning curve, so longer time was required in their first ten cases than in the rest. The idea of preserving muscles and tendons and absence of own experience in this approach made us to be carefully with the method of dissection, lengthening surgery time. All that measures applied in the present report have given 6-week HHS and visual analog pain scores significantly better than in posterior approaches (standard and mini-incision). This experience agrees the reports of Kim (Kim, 2006) and Ogonda (Ogonda et al., 2005) as mini-incision posterior approach implies direct muscle transection and remarks the difference between a small-incision and a tissue sparing surgery.

Minimally invasive techniques require some training and experience in hip surgery, especially for cup placement and femoral exposure. We verified our complications with the use of these techniques and how complications rate changed over time related to surgeons' experience. Of course this is a descriptive not comparative study within all surgeries done by a reduced group of surgeons, so complication rates may not be widespread.

Intraoperative major trochanteric fractures seen in our series related to femoral exposure didn't need fixation in group C as abductor mechanism was not damage. No restrictions were placed on patients postoperatively and no loss of strength, disturbance of gait or pain was notice with these trochanteric avulsions at latest follow-up. Better understanding of the tension applied on the femur and improving in our superior capsular release during exposure resolved this problem. Beside these facts, the stem we have used in group C and some hips of group B (quadra, Medacta®, IT) has a wide proximal section that requires invasion of the inner part of the major trochanter and places it at risk of fracture. On the opposite major throchanteric fractures of group A and B were fixed with cerclage band and gait restrictions were used though not affecting outcomes.

Proximal femoral perforations due to hard reaming of the proximal femur, mainly in muscular male patients with a short varus femoral neck, were our more frequent obstacle to get an accurate stem placement with minimally invasive procedures, mainly in AMIS group. Sariali (Sariali et al., 2008) reported 7 falses reamings of the proximal femur, all noted intra-operatively and without consequences. We noticed this complication in difficult femoral exposures that did not let external rotation and lateral displacement of the proximal femur. All femoral perforations occurred in our learning curve in muscle male patients with severe flexion contractures and have been avoided by improving our technique during femoral broaching. A more horizontal insertion angle of the starting broach is required in these cases for femoral reaming. Careful exposure of the proximal femur and enough releasing of the posterior capsule and pubo-femoral ligament must be done to move the femur in front of the incision.

Periprosthetic fracture and femoral shaft fracture happened after adjusting the bigger stem to a Dorr type C femur and they were detected and resolved intraoperative. We don't agree the idea of higher prevalence of varus stem in minimally invasive procedures (Bernasek et al., 2010) as we have not found outliers in our series (Hart et al., 2005). Cup placement in anterior hip access is another challenge to surgeons familiarized with posterior incision as the pelvis tilt in fracture table. Cup dislodgment reported was a mistake of the surgeon and not a real complication of the technique as he felt self-confident with the acetabulum purchase without testing the grip of the cup.

Rapid early return to function related to minimally invasive surgery (Duwelius & Dorr, 2008; Khan et al., 2006; Seng et al., 2009) has been reported in many papers but these techniques have shown increase complications, especially with the two-incision technique (Desser et al., 2010; Pagnano et al., 2005; Tanavalee et al., 2006). Mini-posterior and direct anterior approach report show rapid recovery function for patients (Duwelius & Dorr, 2008; Klausmeier et al., 2010; Lin et al., 2007; Mardones et al., 2005; Procyk, 2007; Stehlík et al., 2008) but these were limited to the early experience of a few surgeons.

Medical complications encountered in our series were similar to other large series of THAs (Clohisy & Harris, 1999; Duwellius et al., 2007). Paresthesias of the lateral aspect of the thigh (group C) were observed in four cases as we place the incision two finger breadths lateral from ASIS to avoid injuring of the lateral femoral cutaneous nerve.

We can conclude that minimally invasive procedures confer rapid functional recovery of the hip (Bhandari et al., 2009; Fink et al., 2010; Lin et al., 2007; Matta et al., 2005; Pospischill et al., 2010; Varela et al., 2010) and our data suggest that after an education and training schedule for hip experienced surgeons, they could be a safe and reproducible technique. Efforts should focus on how to prevent complications particularly during the learning curve. Moreover, a new spatial guidance for cup and stem placement in anterior hip access should be assumed by surgeons used to lateral and posterior approaches.

5. References

Barton C, Kim PR. Complications of the direct anterior approach for total hip arthroplasty. Orthop Clin North Am 2009; 40 (3): 371- 5

Berend KR, Lombardi AV Jr., Seng BE, Adams JB. Enhanced early outcomes with the anterior supine intermuscular approach in primary total hip arthroplasty. J Bone Joint Surg Am 2009; 91 Suppl 6: 107-20

Berger R, Jacobs JJ, Meneghini RM et al. Rapid rehabilitation and recovery with minimally invasive total hip arthroplasty. Clin Orthop Relat Res 2004; 429: 239-47

Bernasek TL, Lee WS, Lee HJ, Lee JS, Kim KH, Yang JJ. Minimally invasive primary THA: anterolateral intermuscular approach versus lateral transmuscular approach. Arch Orthop Trauma Surg. 2010 Nov; 130(11): 1349-54. Epub 2010 Jan 13

Berry DJ, von Knoch M, Schleck CD, et al. The cumulative long-term risk of dislocation after primary Charnley total hip arthroplasty. J Bone Joint Surg 2004; 86A (1): 9-14

Bhandari M, Matta JM, Dodgin D, Clark C, Kregor P, Bradley G, Little L. Outcomes following the single incision anterior approach to total hip arthroplasty: a multicenter observational study. Orthop Clin North Am. 2009; 40: 329-42

Clohisy JC, Harris WH. The Harris-Galante porous coated acetabular component with screw fixation: an average ten-year follow-up study. J Bone Joint Sur Am 1999; 81: 66-73

D'Arrigo C, Speranza A, Monaco E, Carcangiu A, Ferretti A. Learning curve in tissue sparing total hip replacement: comparison between different approaches. J Orthopaed Traumatol (2009) 10:47–54

De Verteuil R, Imamura M, Zhu S, Glazener C, Fraser C, Munro N, Hutchison J, Grant A, Coyle D, Coyle K, Vale L. A systematic review of the clinical effectiveness and cost-effectiveness and economic modelling of minimal incision total hip replacement approaches in the management of arthritic disease of the hip. Health Technol Assess. 2008 Jun; 12(26): iii-iv, ix-223.

Desser DR, Mitrick MF, Ulrich SD, Delanois RE, Mont MA. Total hip arthroplasty: comparion of two-incision and standart techniques at an AOA-accredited community hospital. J Am Osteopath Assoc. 2010; 110 (1): 12-5

Duncan CP (2006) Minimally invasive or limited incision hip replacement classification. In: Proceedings, MIS meet CAOS symposium, Scottsdale, pp 26–28

Duwelius PJ, Dorr LD. Minimally invasive total hip arthroplasty: an overview of the results. Instr Course Lect. 2008; 57: 215-22

Duwellius PJ, Burkhart RL, Hayhurst JO, Moller H, Butler JB. Comparison of the 2-incision and mini-incision posterior total hip arthroplasty technique: a retrospective match-pair controlled study. J Arthroplasty 2007; 22: 48-56

Fink B, Mittelstaedt A, Schulz MS, Sebena P, Singer J. Comparison of a minimally invasive posterior approach and the standard posterior approach for total hip arthroplasty A prospective and comparative study. J Orthop Surg Res. 2010 Jul 27; 5: 46

Goosen JH, Kollen BJ, Castelein RM, Kuipers BM, Verheyen CC. Minimally invasive versus classic procedures in total hip arthroplasty: a double-blind randomized controlled trial. Clin Orthop Relat Res. 2011 Jan; 469(1): 200-8. Epub 2010 Mar 30

Hart R, Stipcák V, Janecek M, Visna P. Component position following total hip arthroplasty through a miniinvasive posterolateral approach. Acta Orthop Belg. 2005 Feb; 71(1): 60-4

He XH, Tay SS, Ling EA (1988) Sensory nerve endings in monkey hip joint capsule: a morphological investigation. Clin Anat 11(2): 81–85

Heithoff BE, Callaghan JJ, Goetz DD, et al. Dislocation after total hip arthroplasty: a single surgeon's experience. Orthop Clin North Am 2001; 32(4): 587-91

Judet T. Revolution, progression or illusion. Does minimally invasive surgery exist for hip arthroplasty. Interact Surg; 2006; 1: 3-4

Khan RJ, Fick D, Khoo P, Yao F, Nivbrant B, Wood D. Less invasive total hip arthroplasty: description of a new technique. J Arthroplasty 2006 Oct; 21(7): 1038-46

Kim YH. Comparison of primary total hip arthroplasties performed with a minimally invasive technique or standart technique. J Arthroplasty 2006; 21: 1092-8

Klausmeier V, Lugade V, Jewett BA, Collis DK, Chou LS. Is there faster recovery with an anterior or anterolateral THA? A pilot study. Clin Orthop Relat Res. 2010 Feb; 468(2): 533-41. Epub 2009 Sep 10

Lamontagne M, Varin D, Beaulé PE. Does the anterior approach for total hip arthroplasty better restore stair climbing gait mechanics? J Orthop Res 2011 Mar 15. doi: 10.1002/jor.21392. [Epub ahead of print]

Laude F. Total hip arthroplasty through an anterior Hueter minimally invasive approach. Interact Surg 2006; 1: 5-11

Lewinnek GE, Lewis JL, Tarr R, t al. Dislocations after total hip-replacement arthroplasties. J Bone Jt Surg 1978; 60A: 217-20

Lin DH, Jan MH, Liu TK, Lin YF, Hou SM. Effects of anterolateral minimally invasive surgery in total hip arthroplasty on hip muscle strength, walking speed, and functional score. J Arthroplasty. 2007 Dec; 22(8): 1187-92

Lugade V, Wu A, Jewett B, Collis D, Chou LS. Gait asymmetry following an anterior and anterolateral approach to total hip arthroplasty. Clin Biomech (Bristol, Avon). 2010 Aug;25(7): 675-80. Epub 2010 Jun 9

Maffiuletti NA, Impellizzeri FM, Widler K, Bizzini M, Kain MS, Munzinger U, Leunig M. Spatiotemporal parameters of gait after total hip replacement: anterior versus posterior approach. Orthop Clin North Am. 2009 Jul; 40(3): 407-15

Mardones R, Pagnano MW, Nemarish JP, et al. Muscle damage after total hip arthroplasty done with two-incision and mini-posterior techniques. Clin Orthop 2005; 441: 63-7

Mast NH, Laude F. Revision total hip arthroplasty performed through the Hueter interval. J Bone Joint Surg Am. 2011 May;93 Suppl 2:143-8

Matta JM, Shahrdar C, Ferguson T. Single-incision anterior approach for total hip arthroplasty on an orthopaedic fracture table. Clin Orthop Relat Res 2005; 441: 115-24

Matziolis D, Wassilew G, Strube P, Matziolis G, Perka C. Differences in muscle trauma quantifiable in the laboratory between the minimally invasive anterolateral and transgluteal approach. Arch Orthop Trauma Surg. 2011 May; 131(5): 651-5. Epub 2010 Oct 17

Mazoochian F, Weber P, Schramm S, Utzschneider S, Fottner A, Jansson V. Minimally invasive total hip arthroplasty: a randomized controlled prospective trial. Arch Orthop Trauma Surg. 2009 Dec; 129(12): 1633-9. Epub 2009 May 8

Meneghini RM, Pagnanno MW, Trousdale RT, et al. Muscle damage during MIS total hip arthroplasty: Smith-Petersen versus posterior approach. Clin Orthop Relat Res 2005; 453: 292-8

Morris MJ, Berend KR, Lombardi AV Jr. Hemostasis in anterior supine intermuscular total hip arthroplasty: pilot study comparing standart electrocautery and a bipolar sealer. Surg Technol Int 2010; 20: 352-6

Müller M, Tohtz S, Dewey M, Springer I, Perka C. Muscle trauma in primary total hip arthroplasty depending on age, BMI, and surgical approach : Minimally invasive anterolateral versus modified direct lateral approach. Orthopade. 2011 Mar; 40(3): 217-223

Nakata K, Nishikawa M, Yamamoto K, Hirota S, Yoshikawa H. A clinical comparative study of the direct anterior with mini-posterior approach: two consecutive series. J Arthroplasty 2009 Aug; 24(5): 698-704. Epub 2008 Jun 13

Ogonda L, Wilson R, Archibold P, et al. A minimally-incision technique in total hip arthroplasty does not improve early postoperative outcomes. J Bone Joint Surg Am 2005; 87: 701-10

Pagnano MW, Leone J, Lewallen DG, Hanssen AD. Two-incision THA had modest outcomes and some substantial complications. Clin Orthop Relat Res 2005; 441: 86-90

Palieri G, Vetrano M, Mangone M, Cereti M, Bemporad J, Roselli G, D'Arrigo C, Speranza A, Vulpiani MC, Ferretti A. Surgical access and damage extent after total hip arthroplasty influence early gait pattern and guide rehabilitation treatment. Eur J Phys Rehabil Med. 2011 Mar; 47(1): 9-17. Epub 2010 Oct 8

Peters CL, McPherson E, Jackson JD, et al. Reduction in early dislocation rate with large-diameter femoral heads un primary total hip arthroplasty. J Arthroplasty 2007; 22 (6 Suppl-2) 140-4

Pospischill M, Kranzl A, Attwenger B, Knahr K. Minimally invasive compared with traditional transgluteal approach for total hip arthroplasty: a comparative gait analysis. J Bone Joint Surg Am. 2010 Feb; 92(2): 328-37

Procyk S. Initial results with a mini-posterior approach for total hip arthroplasty. Int Orthop. 2007 Aug; 31 Suppl 1: S17-20

Roy L, Laflamme GY, Carrier M, Kim PR, Leduc S. A randomised clinical trial comparing minimally invasive surgery to conventional approach for endoprosthesis in elderly patients with hip fractures. Injury. 2010 Apr; 41(4): 365-9. Epub 2009 Nov 1

Sariali E, Leonard P, Marnoudy P. Dislocation after total hip arthroplasty using Hueter anterior approach. J Arhroplasty 2008; 23: 266-72

Sculco TP, Boettner F. Minimally invasive total hip arthroplasty: the posterior approach. Instr Course Lect. 2006; 55: 205-14

Sculco TP. Minimally invasive total hip arthroplasty. In the affirmative. J Arthroplasty 2004; 19 (4 Suppl 1): 78-80

Seng BE, Berend KR, Ajluni AF, Lombardi AV Jr. Anterior-supine minimally invasive total hip arthroplasty: defining the learning curve. Orthop Clin North Am. 2009 Jul; 40(3): 343-50

Siguier T, Siguier M, Brumpt B. Mini-incision anterior approach does not increase dislocation rate: a study of 1307 total hip replacement. Clin Orthop Relat Res 2004; 426: 164-73

Stehlík J, Musil D, Held M, Stárek M. Minimally invasive total hip replacement--one-year results. Acta Chir Orthop Traumatol Cech. 2008 Aug; 75(4): 262-70

Sugano N, Takao M, Sakai T, Nishii T, Miki H, Nakamura N. Comparison of mini-incision total hip arthroplasty through an anterior approach and a posterior approach using navigation. Orthop Clin North Am. 2009 Jul; 40(3): 365-70

Tanavalee A, Jaruwannapong S, Yuktanandana P, Itiravivong P. Early outcomes following minimally invasive total hip arthroplasty using a two-incision approach versus a mini-posterior approach. Hip Int 2006; 16 Suppl 4: 17-22

Vail TP, Callaghan JJ. Minimal incision total hip arthroplasty. J Am Acad Orthop Surg. 2007 Dec; 15(12): 707-15

Varela Egocheaga JR, Suárez-Suárez MÁ, Fernández-Villán M, González-Sastre V, Varela-Gómez JR, Murcia-Mazón A. Minimally invasive posterior approach in total hip arthroplasty. Prospective randomised trial. An Sist Sanit Navar. 2010 May-Aug; 33(2): 133-43

Waldman BJ. Advancements in minimally invasive total hip arthroplasty. Orthopaedics 2003; 26 (8 Suppl): s 833-6

Wojciechowski O, Kusz D. Kopec K et al. Minimally invasive approaches in total hip arthroplasty. Orthop Traumatol Rehabil 2007; 9(1): 1-7

Zati A, Degli Espoosti S, Spagnoletti C et al (1997) Does total hip arthroplasty mean sensorial and proprioceptive lesion? A clinical study. Chir Organi Mov 82(3): 239-247

3

Degenerative Hip Joint Pain – The Non-Arthroplasty Surgical Options

Ahmed Alghamdi and Martin Lavigne
Université de Montréal
Canada

1. Introduction

Degenerative Hip Joint Pain (DHJP) is a major cause of functional limitation in both young active and old sedentary patients. Total hip arthroplasty (THA) is one of the most successful surgical procedures performed in orthopaedics. Sir John Charnley introduced the concept of low friction arthroplasty for end stage hip arthritis. The rewarding result of this procedure makes THA the gold standard for the treatment of end stage degenerative hip disease. In a recent retrospective study to establish the implant survivorship after THA in young patient at 25 years follow up, up to 89% (80%-98%) survivorship was reported among patients who were diagnosed with developmental dysplasia, 85% (77%-93%) in patients diagnosed with rheumatoid arthritis and 74% (61%-87%) in patients group with idiopathic degenerative arthritis of the hip[1]. Despite improved surgical technique, implant biomaterial and prosthesis design, complications such as recurrent dislocation, osteolysis and loosening still exist. Failure of THA may present with particular problems when revision arthroplasty is needed in young patient, which makes hip joint preservation techniques still actual in this population (hip arthroscopy, surgical dislocation with osteochondroplasty, periacetabular osteotomy, proximal femur osteotomy), and put back on track older surgical procedures such as hip fusion or resection arthroplasty for certain rare indications.

2. Evaluation of painful hip joint

Evaluation of painful hip joint starts with history and physical examination followed by imaging study and laboratory investigation, as needed. Patient with DHJP presents with acute or insidious onset pain, usually with a recurring pattern. It is critical to differentiate sources of hip pain originating from intra-articular pathology from those secondary to extra articular pathology. Intra-articular pathology usually causes deep-seated pain, localized in the anterior groin or inguinal region, although pain of intra-articular origin may be felt at any area around the hip joint. Individuals with symptoms secondary to Femoroacetabular impingements (FAI) might indicate the location of pain by gripping the lateral hip, just above the greater trochanter, between the abducted thumb and index finger. This is known as C-sign[2]. Other symptoms of intra-articular pathology include catching, popping and locking, although those symptoms may represent a misinterpretation of extra-articular conditions such as snapping of the psoas tendon or of the tensor fascia lata.

The pain is usually aggravated by weight bearing, going upstairs, and prolonged seating with hip flexion and adduction as in limited seat space, such as a car seat.

Extra-articular pathology will cause pain mostly in the pubic area, lateral trochanter region, buttock region, or posterior thigh. Referred pain from spine or vascular claudication should be ruled out. Pelvic pathology and anterior abdominal wall hernia might cause pain in the groin region.

Physical examination starts with inspection of the patient gait while getting into the office. A limp, Trendelenburg lurch and poor trunk balance should be looked for[3]. Inspection may disclose pelvis malposition, joint contractures or limb inequality. The foot progression angle should be observed. The patient should sit for history taking. After history, the patient should lay supine on the examination table. Ligament laxity can be tested. Log roll the limb to elicit any pain secondary to intra-articular pathology by rotating the femoral head in the acetabulum. Bony prominences, muscles and tendons around the hip joint, along with, the sciatic nerve and bursa overlying the greater trochanter are then palpated. Anterior abdominal wall examination and groin hernia test should be done. The spine, sacroiliac joint and the knee should also be examined. A complete neurovascular assessment of the limb involved should then be performed. Ranges of motion should be done both actively and passively (Table 1).

Range of motion	Value
Flexion	110-120
Extension	10-15
Abduction	30-50
Adduction	20-30
External rotation at 90 degree	40-60
Internal rotation at 90 degree	30-40

Table 1. Hip range of motion

Special test:
- **Anterior labral stress test:** while the patient in supine position, takes the patients leg into flexion, adduction, and slight internal rotation to compress the anterior part of the labrum. A positive test has occurred if the pain has been reproduced and implies an anterior superior tear. Other clinical finding to look for would be crepitus, popping, clicking.
- **Posterior labral stress test:** patient lay in a prone position, and then the examiner will take the patients leg into passive hyperextension, abduction and external rotation. If this motion elicits the pain, a positive test has occurred secondary to posterior tear.
- **Anterior impingement test:** Passive combination of flexion, adduction and internal rotation will cause pain in the anterior groin, which may suggest the presence of FAI.
- **Posterior impingement test:** hyperextension and external rotation will cause posterior impingement and pain, although pain in this position might be secondary to instability.
- **Ober's test:** The patient is positioned in lateral decubitus with the affected side up. The examiner will stabilize the pelvis from the back and hold the leg in neutral rotation and abduction with the knee in 90 degrees of flexion. The hip is then extended and slowly adducted down towards the table. The knee will not reach the examination table because of restricted adduction due to the tight iliotibial band. Lateral knee pain might occur.

- **Snapping test:** Patient can be asked to reproduce the snapping. An audible snap tends to occur more frequently with internal coxa saltans (psoas snapping on the pubic eminence), and can be reproduced when the hip is actively extended from a flexed and abducted hip position. A palpable sapping on the lateral aspect of the hip suggests external coxa saltans (usually tight of thickened iliotibial band sliding over the greater trochanter). Patient can reproduce external snapping while performing cycling move in lateral decubitus. Palpation over the GT may cause tenderness.
- **The Trendelenburg test** should be performed to rule out gluteus medius weakness.
- **Thomas test:** The patient lay supine on the examination table and hold one knee in direction of his chest, while the other leg remains extended. Positive Thomas test occur when the patient cannot keep the opposing leg extended secondary to the hip fixed flexion contraction.

Imaging study: [4]

- *Anteroposterior (AP) pelvis view:* Standard pelvic view can be taken with the patient supine, or preferably standing. The coccyx should be centered 2-3 cm above the symphisis pubis. Both obturator foramens should look symmetrical.

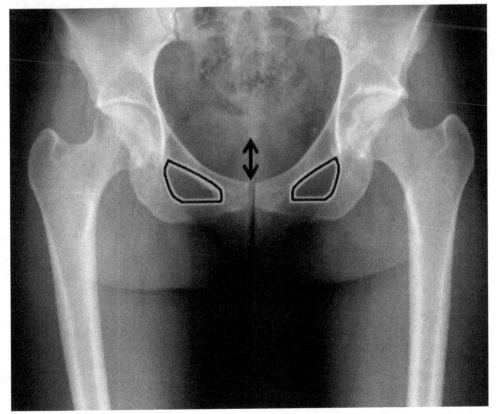

Fig. 1. AP pelvic view, centered view; symmetric obturator foramina, centered coccyx with 2-3 cm distance above the pubic symphisis.

- Lateral views of the hip:
  - *Frog leg lateral:* mostly a view of the proximal femur
  - *Cross table lateral:* view the acetabulum and proximal femur
  - *Dunn 45/90:* specific view of anterior femoral head-neck junction. This view can be taken with the hip at 45 or 90 degree of flexion.
  - *False profile:* for measuring anterior acetabular coverage

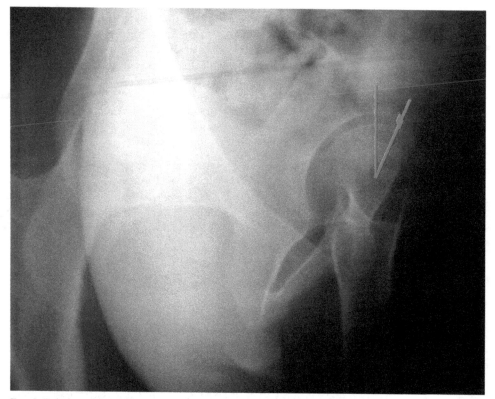

Fig. 2. False-profile view, the anterior centre-edge (VCA) angle quantifies the anterior cover of the femoral head, and angles of less than 20° are considered abnormal.

- *AP hip view:* the x-ray beam is centered on the hip joint. Not reliable for cross over sign.
- *Computer Tomography (CT) scans:* with 3-D reconstruction, can be more accurate for preoperative impingement evaluation or other deformation of acetabulum or femur.
- *Magnetic resonance imaging (MRI) scan:* good diagnostic tool for both soft tissue and bone strucutre. Intra-articular contrast injection can be use for further evaluation of labrum. Alpha angle of Notzli was described on a specific MRI view, although it is currently measured on different radiographic modalities[5].
- *Ultrasound scan:* can provide dynamic evaluation. It can be used as therapeutic tool as well[6].
- *Bone scan:* usually non specific
- *Bursography:* can be used for snapping hip.

3. Hip arthroscopy

The first recorded attempt of arthroscopic visualization of the hip joint is attributed to Michael Burman in 1930. The limited indications of hip arthroscopy at that time and the anatomic constraints of the hip joint with suboptimal equipment design have limited the use of hip arthroscopy for long time. However with improved hip arthroscopy tools, the indications for hip arthroscopy continue to evolve. Currently, many clinical issues related to the hip joint and the surrounding tissue can be treated with hip arthroscopy. Degenerative hip conditions that can be treated with hip arthroscopy are listed in Table 2.

Degenerative Indications	Non-Degenerative indications
• Labral Lesions • Chondral injuries • FAI • Degenerative arthritis	• Loose bodies (traumatic or synovial chondomatosis) • Sepsis • Synovial disease • Instability • Coxa Sultan (extern or intern)

Table 2. Conditions treated with hip arthroscopy

3.1.1 Labral lesions

The etiology of labral tear is traumatic, degenerative, idiopathic or congenital. Labral pathology can also be classified based on location (anterior, superolateral, posterior). Anterior labral tears are the most common form in the western population, accounting for 90% of cases. Degenerative labral tears are more and more frequently felt to result from FAI and usually starts in the avascular (water-shield) white zone of the labral structure. In this zone, there is low chance of successful healing of the labral tear with conservative treatment. Labral tears may cause pain and microinstability of the hip joint. They also may increase friction within the joint and the strain within the articular cartilage; thereby possibly untreated lesion will result in accelerated degeneration of the joint. In FAI, persisting conflict between femoral neck and acetabulum will lead to chondral delamination and thinning, further the labral tear, paralabral cyst and ultimately, degenerative osteoarthritis

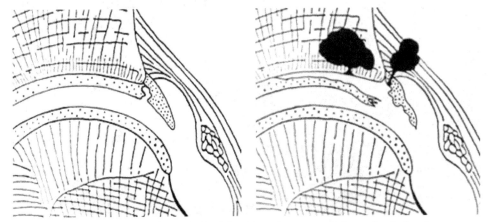

Fig. 3. Labral Tear begins at the articular labral junction, termed the *watershed region*. Progressive labral degenerations result in paralabral cysts and articular cartilage damage.

of the involved joint. With hip arthroscopy, the labrum can be debrided, resected, repaired or reconstructed.

3.1.2 Femoroacetabular impingement (FAI)

This is a descriptive diagnosis characterized by combined clinical features and pathomorphological findings that can result in degenerative changes. The patient's pathomorphology is characterized by either cam lesion, pincer lesion or a combination of both. Mechanical abutment of cam lesion commonly causes pathological changes starting with focal, deep chondral delamination in the anterolateral (superolateral) region of the acetabulum. Separation of the labrum-chondral junction will allow the synovial fluid to extravasate to the subchondral bone or para-labral region creating intra osseous or para-labral cyst (Figure 3). Leverage of head-cam lesion against the acetabulum with extreme range of motion can result in contre-coup lesion in posterinferior acetabulum [7]. Leading to global degenerative changes.

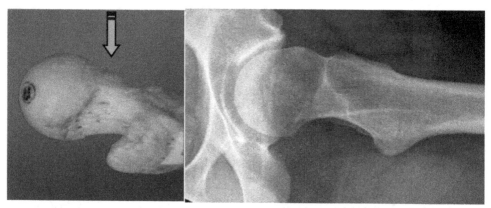

Fig. 4. Cam lesion as seen in skeletonized specimen and frog leg lateral view.

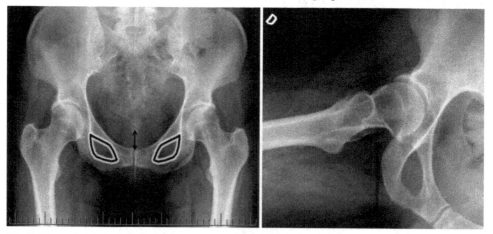

Fig. 5. Pincer Lesion, global over-coverage and labral calcification in 45 years old female. Notice the relatively minor degenerative changes on the anterior femoral head neck junction.

The pincer lesion will cause a crush-type injury of the labrum and progressive degenerative changes with minimal damage to the articular cartilage of the acetabulum.

Indication of hip arthroscopy in this setting is symptomatic FAI with concomitant labral and or cartilage lesion. The labrum is addressed as mentioned in the previous section, while the cartilage damage is addressed by debridement or micro fracture of the underlying subchondral bone. The osseous abnormalities are treated with an osteochondroplasty and acetabuloplasty as needed.

3.1.3 Degenerative arthritis

Arthroscopic intervention in early hip joint degeneration may relieve pain and others associated symptoms (i.e. catching, locking and range of motion limitation). However, as seen with knee arthroscopy, it provides little benefit on the long term and thus represents a limited indication for hip arthroscopy. Hip arthroscopy in this clinical scenario will provide limited role through removal of loose bodies, debridement of degenerative chondral or labral tears and subtotal synovectomy. Capsular release and osteophyte excision might improve the hip range of motion.

Before attempting hip arthroscopy for advance degenerative changes, patient needs to know the limitation of such procedure. The patient are less likely to benefit from hip arthroscopy when joint space is less than 50% of normal, with pain at rest, functionally depleting limitation of hip range of motion or pre-operative Harris Hip Score (HHS) of less than 60.

3.2 Surgical technique

Under general, spinal or combined anesthesia, the patient is positioned supine or in lateral decubitus according to the surgeon's preference. This section will only address the hip arthroscopy while the patient on supine position. A well-padded perineal post will be used to protect the pubis and provide counter traction force during distraction of the hip joint. The foot should also be well-padded befor connecting the foot attachments. Distraction of the hip joint is gently performed with the hip slightly flexed in neutral abduction and rotation until approximately 8 mm of joint space is achieved. Multiple portals can be used to visualize both central (articular surfaces) and peripheral (extra articular) compartments of the hip joint. Common portals used are anterior, anterolateral and posterolateral in relation to the Greater Trochanter (GT). Fluoroscopic views should be used during portal preparation to ensure enough joint distraction and to avoid labral penetration. The 70-degree lens is used most of the time. Labral tear, cartilage damage or over coverage can be treated as described above. Inspection of the peripheral compartment and excision of the cam lesion can be done without traction with the use of fluoroscopy x-ray to guide precise cam lesion excision. Dynamic assessment is helpful to assess the relief of FAI.

3.3 Postoperative rehabilitation

After arthroscopic osteochondroplasty and labral debridement, full weight bearing will be permitted, unless micro fractures were performed, in which case toe touch weight bearing is recommended for 6-8 weeks. Aggressive active-passive range of motion and proprioception exercise will be started early post operative. High impact sport is not allowed for 2 months post femoral neck osteoplasty.

3.4 Complications
Complications occur in 0.5% to 5% of patients and are most often related to the required distraction of the hip joint [8]. Sciatic, femoral or pudendal nerve palsy can result from prolonged traction time. Nerve injury tends to be transient neuropraxia, which completely resolve spontaneously in few weeks. A well-padded post should prevent perineal tear and pudendal nerve injury. Bleeding and lateral femoral cutaneous nerve injury can occur during portal placement. Postoperative persistent secondary to trochanteric bursitis, intra-articular capsular adhesion (especially between the capsule and repaired labrum, or between the capsule and anterior neck) may occur. Femoral neck fracture, avascular necrosis of the femoral head, and under or over resections of cam lesion can be a mode of failure. Instrumental breakage rarely happen, but sometimes requires open arthrotomy to remove the broken fragment. Incidence of deep venous thrombosis ranges from 0 to 3.7% in various retrospective clinical reports[9].

3.5 Results of arthroscopic FAI surgery
Hip arthroscopy for the treatment of FAI has only been used recently. Philippon et al studied 45 professional athletes at 1.6 years (6 months to 5.5 years) follow up. 93% of patients returned to professional competition, but only 78% remained active in professional sport at final follow up[10].

Sampson et al analyzed the results of 183 patients (194 hips) with positive impingement sign at preoperative assessment at maximum follow up of 29 months. 95% of the patients showed no sign of impingement at one year after surgery[11].

Byrd et al found an improvement of Harris Hip Score (HHS) from baseline of 20 points (range 17 to 60 point), which was reported in 83% of patients at 1 year follow up[12].

Another study reported by Philippon et al analyzed 112 patients at mean follow up of 2.3 years. The HHS improved from 58 to 84.3 in those patients with FAI associated with labral and chondral pathology. However, 8.9% of the patient underwent THA at mean follow up of 16 months[13].

4. Combined limited open arthrotomy and hip arthroscopy

Combined limited open arthrotomy and hip arthroscopy can be utilized to treat symptomatic anterolateral FAI: the hip arthroscopy will focus on any labral pathology and allow microfracturing for acetabular chondral damage. The limited arthrotomy approach will allow easy access to the pathologic part of the femoral head neck junction.

4.1 Surgical technique
Patient is positioned supine, exactly the same as described in previous section. After arthroscopic treatment of labral and chondral lesions, the traction is released. Anterior or anterolateral approach can be performed. We prefer a modified Watson-Jones approach, which allow better visualization of the anterolateral and posterolateral aspect of head neck junction. The 8-10 cm incision starts 2-3 cm distal and 2-3 cm lateral to the Anterior Superior Iliac Spine (ASIS) directed distally and laterally toward the anterior tip of GT. Subcutaneous dissection is carried down to the fascia lata. The interval between Tensor Fascia Lata (TFL) and Gluteus Medius (GM) muscles can be identified just anterior to the GT after incising the fascia. The GM is retracted posteriorly while the TFL is retracted anteromedialy. The rectus femoris tendon is identified and the hip joint capsule exposed. A T-shaped capsulotomy is

performed with care to prevent injury of the labrum. Spiked tip retractors can be placed intracapsular anterior and posterior around the rim of the acetabulum which will allow safe dynamic assessment of the hip joint. We use a high-speed burr to resect the cam lesion on the anterolateral femoral neck then ensure effective resection by using intraoperative fluoroscopy and dynamic assessment of the hip joint. Removing all bone debris and minimizing muscle damage can play significant role in reducing the incidence of Heterotopic Ossification (HO). Capsular and fascia lata closure are performed at the end of the procedure.

4.2 Postoperative care

Weight bearing as tolerated is permitted early post operatively. Contact sport is not allowed for at least 2-3 months. Active and passive range of motion along with unrestricted strengthening is allowed. However, when rectus femoris tendon is violated, then restrictions will be applied on active straight leg raise (SLR) for 6 weeks. Subcutaneous low molecular weight heparin is given for 10 days.

4.3 Complications
1. Deep venous thromboses and thromboembolic disease.
2. Neurovascular injury.
3. Infection.
4. Femoral neck fracture.
5. HO.
6. Femoral head avascular necrosis (AVN)
7. Complications related to hip arthroscopy procedure.

4.4 Results

Lincoln et al reported a significant difference between the mean Harris hip score preoperatively and that at last follow-up (from 63.8 to 76.1) of 16 hips treated using a modified Heuter anterior approach combined with adjunctive hip arthroscopy.

Clohisy et al reported the results of combined arthroscopy and limited open osteochondroplasty for anterior FAI in 35 patients. HHS improved from 63.8 to 87.4 at minimum follow up of 2 years. No fracture of the femoral neck or AVN of the femoral head was reported[14].

Pierannunzii et al found that the mean HHS improved from 74.4 to 85.3 in 8 patients at mean follow up of 10 months[15].

5. Surgical dislocation of the hip joint

5.1 Indications

Surgical dislocation of the hip joint for the treatment of FAI is safe when performed with appropriate understanding of the vascular anatomy of the proximal femur. Surgical dislocation of the hip is considered the gold standard procedure for the treatment of FAI, despite the advance of hip arthroscopy technique and the encouraging results of the limited open surgical procedure. Surgical dislocation of the hip is especially indicated with global or posterior impingement requiring acetabular rim trimming, with severe deformity of the proximal femur or when chondral lesions of the femoral head have to be addressed. Patient with no more than mild arthrosis (Tonnis <=2) and age less than 50 years are considered the best candidates for such surgical intervention.

5.2 Contraindications
Advance arthrosis, is a contraindication for this procedure.

5.3 Surgical technique
The patient positioned in lateral decubitus under general or combined general and spinal anesthesia. The pelvis should be stabilized in proper orientation to allow proper evaluation of the acetabular version.

The incision is curvilinear, approximately 20-25 cm in length and centered over the GT curving slightly posteriorly at 20 degree angle. The fascia lata is incised and the interval between TFL and Gluteus Maximus (GMax) is developed to avoid violation of the GMax muscle fibers. The peritrochantric bursa is incised and retracted anteriorly. The greater trochanter, short external rotators, gluteus medius and vastus lateralis should be clearly visualized. The leg is positioned in 20-30 degrees of internal rotation and an oscillating saw is used to create a trigastrics sliding trochanteric osteotomy of 1-1.5cm thicknesses. Next the leg is repositioned in neutral rotation and the gluteus minimus is dissected off the hip capsule from posterior to anterior to allow full mobilization of the trochanteric fragment anteriorly for performing a safe Z-shape capsulotomy, the capsular incision starts at the anterior boarder of the GT and is directed proximally in line with the femoral neck with care

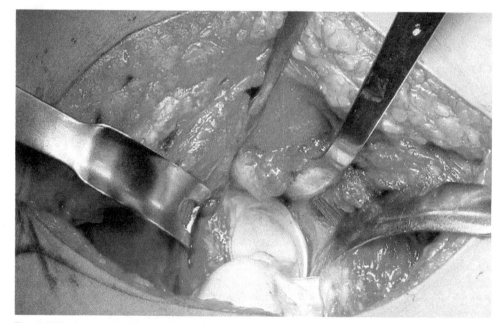

Fig. 6. 360 view provide inspection of the acetabulum, one retractor is impacted above the acetabulum. One retractor hooked on the anterior acetabular rim and a third retractor levers the neck against the incisura acetabuli.

not to injure the labrum. The proximal arm of the capsulotomy runs parallel to the acetabulum posteriorly toward the piriformis tendon, the closest the capsulotomy to the acetabular edge the less likely to risk injuring the lateral epiphyseal branches. The distal arm of the Z-shaped capsulotomy should not extend beyond the lesser trochanter. Distraction force with the use of bone hook with the hip in flexion and external rotation can help dislocating the femoral head. The ligamentum teres can prevent complete dislocation and a curved blunt tip long scissor should be used to cut the ligament if circumferential exposure of the femoral head is required. A straight spiked Hohmann retractor is placed anteriorly around the acetabular rim and a curved Hohmann is placed inferiorly under the transverse ligament to push the femoral head posteriorly. The leg is placed in a sterile bag anteriorly across the table. This will provide 360-degree acetabular exposure for cartilage defects treatment, acetabular rim trimming and labral re-fixation (Figure 6). To treat pathology on the femoral side, the retractors are removed and the head and neck are delivered back into the surgical wound for evaluation and treatment of any head cartilage defect and head-neck junction pathology (Figure 7).

When satisfactory treatment is completed, the femoral head is reduced and the capsule is closed with loose interrupted suture to prevent stretch of retinacular vessels. The greater trochanter fragment should be reduced and fixed with three 3.5mm screws. The fascia lata and overlying skin are closed in layers (Figure 8).

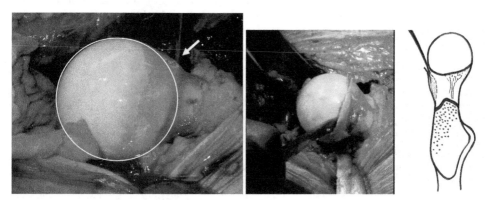

Fig. 7. The hip is flexed, externally rotated and distracted to dislocation of the femoral head. The cam lesion inspected and femoral neck osteoplasty is performed.

5.4 Postoperative care
Patient will be on DVT prophylaxis for 35 days and HO prophylaxis for 2 weeks (Celebrx 200mg twice a day). The patient will be allowed toe touch weight bearing for 6 weeks. Passive range of motion is allowed in all directions, however active abduction and deep flexion beyond 90 degree are not allowed for at least 6 weeks.

5.5 Complications
Complications of the surgical dislocation approach for patients who had had the procedure for multiple differential diagnoses (including Femoroacetabular impingement, Legg-Calve-Perthes disease in a skeletally mature hip, trauma, and deformity following a slipped capital

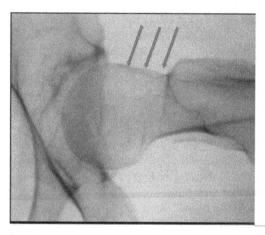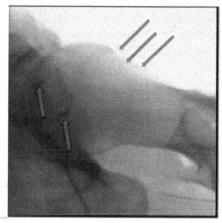

Fig. 8. Preoperative (left) and postoperative (right) lateral views of proximal femur and the acetabulum. Improved head neck offset after excision of the cam lesion. Notice the labral refixation after acetabuloplasty.

femoral epiphysis) were reported by different North American centers that participate in the ANCHOR (Academic Network for Conservational Hip Outcomes Research) group[16]. We listed all possible complications might be anticipated with this procedure, however ANCHOR have reported no cases of osteonecrosis, femoral neck fracture, or any complication leading to long-term morbidity, with the exception of the one sciatic nerve injury, which partially resolved.

1. DVT (0.5%)
2. Infection.
3. Neurovascular injury (permanent and complete major nerve palsy was not reported, however partial sciatic nerve palsy occur in one patient eventually recovered partially).
4. Heterotopic ossification (Brooke I & II 5.3%)[17].
5. Trochanteric fragment displacement and delay union (0.5% require no intervention), or nonunion (rate of 1.8 % that required refixation).
6. Femoral neck fracture
7. AVN
8. Hardware complications: breakage, irritation of surrounding soft tissue (trochanteric bursitis, psoas tendon when prominent medially).
9. Under-correction, or over correction of cam and pincer lesion.
10. Capsular adhesion.

5.6 Results

Retrospective reports demonstrate significant improvement in both radiographic and clinical functional scores.

Murphy et al reported on the surgical dislocation approach for FAI treatment in 23 patients with a mean follow up of 62 months. Preoperative hip scores of Merle d'Aubigné scale were average 13.2 (range, 11-15). THA was performed for 7 patients. Of the surviving 15 hips, the hip scores improved significantly to 16.9 ± 1.35 (range 13-18). No case of AVN was reported[18].

Likewise, Peters et al reported improvement in the mean Harris Hip Score from 70 points preoperatively to 87 points at the time of final follow-up in 29 patients [19].

Beaule et al reported the functional outcome of 34 patients (37 hip) following surgical dislocation to treat cam lesion with mean follow up period of 31.4 years. All activity and functional score demonstrated improved outcome (WOMAC score 61.2 to 81.4, UCLA activity scores 4.8 to 7.5, and mean SF-12 46.4 to 51.2). No osteonecrosis was reported and 9 patients required hardware removal [20].

Espinosa et al found less arthrosis at final follow up in 52 patients (60 hips) when labrum was refixed instead of removed after rim trimming for pincer type impingement. The recovery time and the final clinical and radiographic features favored labral re-fixation[21].

Beck et al reported the mid-term results of surgical dislocation of 19 hips and concluded that this procedure was not suitable for patient with advanced degenerative changes[22]. The same conclusion also reported by Murphy et al [18].

6. Periacetabular osteotomy

Developmental dysplasia of the hip can result in structural instability that exacerbates shearing forces across a limited acetabular cartilage surface area. Ultimately, the abnormal force distribution can result in rim failure and progressive degenerative hip disease[23].

The aim of periacetabular osteotomy is to change the acetabular cavity orientation, thus optimizing the joint mechanics through restoration of joint stability and transformation of *shearing forces* on an oblique acetabular roof to *compressive forces* on a reoriented horizontal acetabular roof.

It was found on long term radiographic follow up that patients with a Center Edge Angle (CEA) less than 16 degrees, acetabular index greater than 15 degrees and femoral head uncoverage more than 30% have higher incidence of osteoarthritis by age 60 [24].

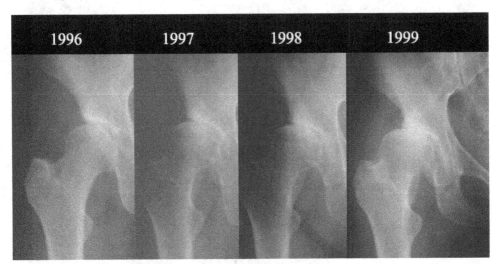

Fig. 9. Natural history of untreated acetabular dysplasia.

Various pelvic osteotomies were proposed to treat symptomatic hip dysplasia. Most of the techniques apply to the infant or adolescents. Salter innominate osteotomy has limited degree of correction in adult hip dysplasia and it dose not solve hip-center lateralization because the acetabular fragment rotation is hinged on a fixed point (symphisis pubis). Double and triple osteotomy provides more freedom for rotation of the osteotomized fragment but since the acetabular fragment is still attached to the sacropelvic ligament, only limited correction angle is possible. This angle of correction can be improved through placing the osteotomy closer to the acetabulum. One disadvantage of this type of osteotomy is the size of acetabular fragment that can cause pelvic narrowing and might interfere with future child bearing in female patient. Spherical periacetabular osteotomy is a highly demanding surgical procedure; it can improve acetabular coverage but can't improve hip-center lateralization because the medial acetabular wall is intact. The osteotomy passes close to the acetabulum capsular attachment, which is considered to be an important source of blood supply to the acetabular bone. Performing a capsulotomy to evaluate intra-articular structure at the remaining time of the osteotomy will jeopardize the acetabular blood supply[25].

Reinhold Ganz initially described Bernese Periacetabular Osteotomy (PAO)[26]. It became widely recognized as an effective osteotomy for the treatment of acetabular dysplasia. Through improved geometric cut around the acetabulum, the polygonal shape acetabular fragment can be reoriented to achieve almost unlimited femoral head coverage and acetabular version as well as allowing control of medialization of the hip-center when needed. The vascular anatomy around the acetabulum is preserved, which allow safe capsulotomy for simultaneous evaluation and treatment of intra-articular pathology.

6.1 Indications

The clinical uses of Bernese PAO in adult patient are indicated in the presence of the following situations:

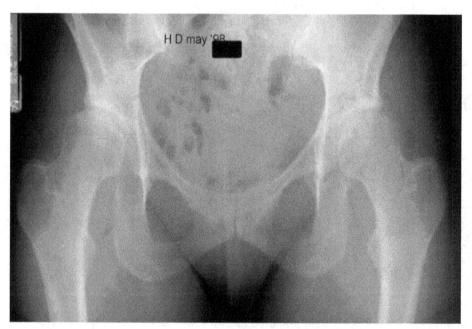

Fig. 10. Bilateral acetabular dysplasia in 17 years old patient.

1. Congruent and symptomatic early hip joint degenerative disease (Tonnis 1).
2. 20-30 degree of hip abduction range of motion.
3. Dysplastic acetabulum with
    a. CEA <20 degree
    b. Tonnis angle >10 degree
4. symptomatic acetabular retroversion without dysplasia can be an indication for PAO, it: Acetabular retroversion can be identified on a standard AP pelvis view (symmetrical obturator foramen and coccyx centered 2-3 cm above the symphisis pubis). The patient radiographic finding will be consistent with acetabulum retroversion if the hip center of rotation is lateral to posterior acetabular rim and the patient have both cross-over sign and ischeal spine sings[27, 28].

6.2 Contraindications
1. Open triradiate cartilage
2. Grade II Tonnis changes and more
3. Incongruent joint
4. Age over 40 has been associated with less favorable outcome in some studies[29, 30].

6.3 Surgical technique
Under general anesthesia, the patient is positioned supine and the limb on the dysplastic acetabulum side is prepped and draped free in sterile fashion. Antibiotics are given before incising the skin. A cell saver is used during this procedure.

A curvilinear incision is starting from the gluteal tubercle on the iliac crest and curved lateral to the ASIS distally for approximately 20 cm. Abdominal external oblique muscle is

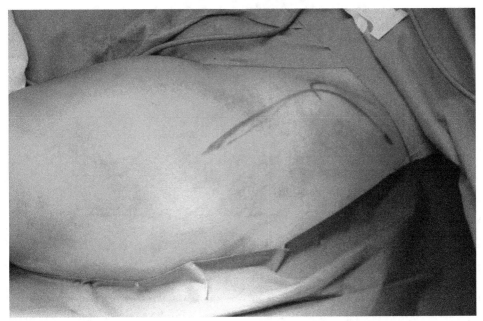

Fig. 11. Curvilinear incision for the anterior approach to perform PAO.

elevated off the internal iliac crest and the interval between TFL and the Sartorius is defined. The ASIS is osteotomized and retracted medially to expose the rectus femoris, which is released from the AIIS. The sartorius and rectus femoris are retracted medially and the TFL is retracted laterally. The ilocapsularis muscle is elevated off the anterior capsule. A spiked Hohmann retractor can be slid over the superior pubic ramus 1.5 cm medial to iliopectineal eminence and serves to retract the medial soft tissue including the psoas and the neurovascular bundle. The medial capsular tissue is freed of soft tissue attachment using long blunt and curved scissors. This provides a window to reach the ischeal tubercle and infracotyloid region, which is also freed of soft tissue attachments.

Four bone cuts are performed to create a polygonal acetabular fragment:

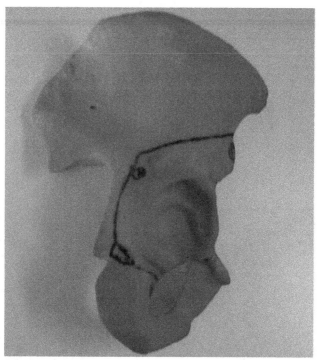

Fig. 12. Polygonal cuts around the acetabulum.

1. Partial ischeal cut using curved Ganz osteotome (avoid sciatic nerve injury by abducting the hip joint)
2. Superior pubic ramus cut using straight osteotome starting medial to iliopectineal eminence (avoid penetrating the joint by aiming 45 degrees medial, away from the acetabulum).
3. Iliac bone cut starting just distal to ASIS toward greater sciatic notch using oscillating saw.
4. The posterior column cut is one centimeter thick and done using both straight and curved osteotome starting off the third cut end with an angle of approximately120 degrees to join the first ischeal cut.

The acetabular fragment should be now free for re-orientation. We use two Schantz screws inserted in the acetabular fragment away from the zone of fixation to accomplish efficient orientation in both abduction and anteversion. Fluoroscopy is used to assess acetabulum version and orientation. The fragment can be allowed to rotate freely around the hip center of rotation. When the desired orientation is achieved, preliminary fixation is obtained with multiple Steinmann pins. True AP pelvic X-ray is done prior final fixation. Multiple screws are used to fix the acetabular fragment. The hip is then taken through full range of motion and if 90-degrees of flexion cannot be achieved, retroversion is corrected or a capsulotomy can be safely done to resolve any intra-articular pathology responsible for impingement.

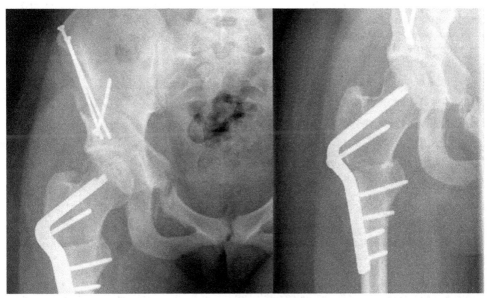

Fig. 13. Postoperative x-ray of the right hip for the same patient presented previously (figure 11) demonstrates combined PAO and proximal femoral osteotomy.

The rectus tendon is reattached to the AIIS using nonabsorbable suture transfixed through drill hole in the iliac bone. The ASIS is fixed with a screw or nonabsorbable suture drilled through the osteotomiesed fragment. A drain is left in place while closure is performed[31].

6.4 Postoperative care
Patients will be on DVT prophylaxis for 35 days. Non-weight bearing is indicated for 6 weeks, and then progressive weight bearing is started when radiographic evidence of healing of the osteotomy. Straight leg raising exercise is delayed for 6 weeks, and the hip joint can be taken through passive range of motion early postoperative.

6.5 Complications
Minor and major complications can occur when doing Bernese PAO. The complexity of the procedure combined with the surgeon learning curve can affect the overall outcome. It was observer that the major complication rate ranged from 6% to 37%[32]. There was a

statistically significant decrease in major complications from 17% to 2.9% when comparing the first 35 cases with the second 35 cases of periacetabular osteotomy performed by one surgeon[33].

The complications reported in literatures include:

1. *General surgical complications:* such as bleeding, DVT, infection and HO
2. *Technique-related complication:* include nerve traction injury to the femoral nerve. Lateral cutaneous nerves of the thigh are involved commonly but usually recover. Sciatic nerve injury is rare. Femoral artery injury or femoral vein thrombosis can occur.
3. *Acetabular-fragment related complications:* include fracture through the posterior column, intra-articular extension of the osteotomy, under or over correction. Delayed union can happen, but nonunion of the acetabular fragment is rare; although nonunion of the superior pubic ramus osteotomy tends to occur more frequently.
4. *Hardware complications:* include joint penetration, fixation failure secondary to broken or migrated screw. Prominent screw can rub against the surrounding tissue leading to painful bursitis.

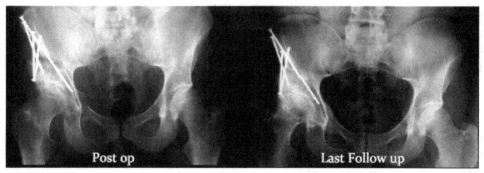

Fig. 14. Progressive degenerative changes lead to failure of PAO.

Ganz et al reported the need for removal of hardware in 17% and HO in 5%, however Trousdale et al reported 33% incidence of HO after PAO. The lateral femorocutaneous nerve is the most commonly injured (30%).[34-36]

6.6 Results

Clohisy et al has made a systematic review of the reported radiographic and clinical results of PAO based on the literatures published up to 2007 with certain inclusion criteria. There were 13 studies with a level of evidence that was generally low (IV). These data derived from various surgeons and institutions indicate PAO can reliably achieve deformity correction. All studies including clinical outcome analysis showed pain relief and improved hip function in the majority of patients at short to midterm follow up. In seven studies, there were correlated between suboptimal clinical results and advanced preoperative osteoarthritis. Failure of the osteotomy and the need to conversion to THA was noted in 0% to 17% of the cases [32].

7. Femoral osteotomy

Various proximal femoral osteotomies were described for different clinical indications. Intertrochanteric Osteotomy (ITO) may be used in adults, although the indications for ITO nowadays are more limited due to the improved outcome of THA. ITO may be useful to provide containment, congruency, coverage or rotational re-alignment of the hip joint through valgus, varus, flexion, extension, rotation or combination of all of these osteotomies. Post-traumatic deformity, rotational malalignment of the lower extremity, coxa valga, slipped capital femoral epiphysis and Legg-Calvé-Perthes disease are clinical conditions where ITO is commonly used.

7.1 Contraindications
1. Advanced degenerative changes
2. Inflammatory arthritis
3. The impossibility of obtaining a congruent joint on functional radiographic views
4. Limited joint range of motion with marked hip stiffness
5. Other relative contra-indications are advanced age, tobacco smoking and morbid obesity.

7.2 Surgical technique
The pre-requisite for a successfully executed ITO is proper pre-operative planning, adequate range of motion and appropriate choice of the fixation device.
A direct lateral approach to the femur is used. The planned osteotomy is performed under fluoroscopic assistance and defined with Steinman pins. A blade plate is used for fixation and the corresponding chisel is inserted in the desired position. The osteotomy is performed with an oscillating saw and can be fixed under compression with a blade plate or condylar plate.

7.3 Postoperative care
DVT prophylaxis is given for 2 weeks, and weight-bearing protection should de respected for 2 months. Passive and active ranges of motion are permitted.

7.4 Postoperative complications
In addition to common surgical complications, AVN and delayed union or non-union of the osteotomy can occur. Over correction or under correction can be a source of patient dissatisfaction. Hardware failure or soft tissue irritation might require removal after fracture healing.

7.5 Results
Multiple clinical studies on the use of proximal femoral osteotomy are reported in the literatures. Haverkamp et al reported the results of 276 patients that had ITO for various indications. The best clinical results at 10 years were achieved when the osteotomy was performed in young patient with posttraumatic deformity (90% success rate at 10 years). Arthritic changes in association with an idiopathic etiology had the worst results with only 50% success rate at final follow up[37].

8. Salvage procedure for degenerative hip joint pain

Salvage surgery, including the Chiari osteotomy and shelf procedures; do not provide coverage of the femoral head by a surface of hyaline cartilage. The hip capsule is interposed between newly formed acetabular roof and femoral head.

- *Chiari Pelvic Osteotomy:* Chiari medial displacement pelvic osteotomy may be used to treat degenerative hip pain in young patient with incongruent hip joint. The osteotomy is performed at 15 degrees superior inclination within the supracetabular iliac bone and the hip joint is displaced medially to improve superior coverage of the femoral head. Excessively low or too high osteotomy cut can give suboptimal clinical result. Sufficient acetabular fragment medial displacement is critical to provide enough femoral head coverage. The superior capsule is used as the articular surface under the displaced ilium. The posterinferior aspect of the hip is spared from disease, as seen on the false-profile roentgenogram. and a reconstructive osteotomy can be performed. Furthermore anterior coverage of the head is difficult to obtain with a medial displacement osteotomy. This procedure relies on fibrocartlage metaplasia of the capsule, results in lower functional outcome compared to other periacetabular osteotomies or THA. One advantage of this type of osteotomy is improving future acetabular component bone fixation[38].
- *Shelf Procedure:* Placing a bone graft in the superolateral region of the acetabulum as a shelf can provide containment and coverage of the femoral head, thus preventing lateral or upward migration of the femoral head. The shelf procedure provides greater lateral coverage but the original steep inclination of the acetabulum persists. The technique can be used as a supplemental procedure with other type of osteotomy and can be performed with a limited incision technique[39].

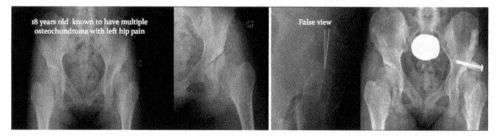

Fig. 15. Shelf procedure.

8.1 Hip fusion (arthrodesis)

Young patients with advanced unilateral degenerative hip changes, secondary to trauma or septic conditions are good candidate for hip fusion. Hip arthrodesis provides better clinical results in young (less than 35) active patient with normal contralateral hip, no pathology in the ipsilateral knee or lower spine and when the hip fusion technique preserves the abductor muscles integrity. Although a valuable option, it has many drawbacks including loss of motion, shortening of the extremity, increased expenditure of energy during walking, and increased stress on the low back and the ipsilateral knee[40].

Several techniques have been described. The femoral head and the acetabulum are denuded of cartilage and the hip is positioned in approximately 30 degrees of flexion, 0 to 5 degrees of adduction and 10 degrees of external rotation. The fixation can be intra articular (screws through the femoral head to the iliac bone), or extra articular (side plate, cobra plate, anterior plate). A trochanteric osteotomy is advisable to preserve the abductor function for future conversion of hip fusion to THA when side plate or cobra plate is used.

The reported clinical results of THA after hip fusion demonstrate a wide spectrum of clinical outcome. Hamadouche et al studies 45 THA performed after hip fusion at a mean follow up of 8.5 years. He reported 91% survival with walking improvement up to 2-3 years after surgery, however, 50% of patients required a cane for walking[41]. Joshi et al found that 79% of the patients had minimal pain with a 96% 10 years survival. The complications reported for the 208 fused hips converted to THA were 8 sciatic nerve and 7 femoral nerve palsies, 28 cases of HO, 5 dislocations and 3 infections[42].

9. Resection arthroplasty

Gathome Girdlestone described the surgical technique of resection arthroplasty of the hip joint to palliate hip condition secondary to chronic infection (i.e. tuberculosis hip infection). This procedure has been widely used to relive pain or to improve the hip range of motion in conditions such as advanced hip degeneration and chronic hip joint infection. Improvement in the treatment of infection, fracture fixation technique and the introduction of prosthetic hip replacement has significantly limited the role of hip resection arthroplasty. The current indications for resection arthroplasty are nonambulatory patient with significant cognitive or neuromuscular condition or patient with chronic prosthesis infection and significant comorbidity that cannot go through complex surgical procedure. After the Girdlestone procedure, patients have significant functional limitations secondary to weak abductor and limb length inequality[43].

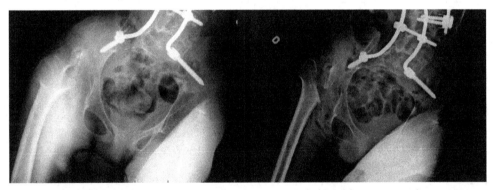

Fig. 16. 21 years old male patient (cerebral palsy patient), his health care provider notice increasing difficulty with perineal hygiene and increasing irritability when diaper changes are attempted. Intertrochanteric resection was performed to improve his hip range of motion and to alleviate his symptoms.

10. Summary

Non-arthroplasty surgical options for treating painful degenerative hip joint conditions are well established surgical procedures. Patient selection and proper preoperative evaluation is critical for successful long-term result. Understanding the indications and the contraindications as well as the limitations and the expected outcome of each procedure is critical during pre operative counseling of the patient about nonarthroplasty surgical option.

11. References

[1] Sochart, D.H. and M.L. Porter, *The long-term results of Charnley low-friction arthroplasty in young patients who have congenital dislocation, degenerative osteoarthrosis, or rheumatoid arthritis.* J Bone Joint Surg Am, 1997. 79(11): p. 1599-617.

[2] Dooley, P.J., *Femoroacetabular impingement syndrome: Nonarthritic hip pain in young adults.* Can Fam Physician, 2008. 54(1): p. 42-7.

[3] Van Iersel, M. and G. Mulley, *What is a waddling gait?* Disability & Rehabilitation, 2004. 26(11): p. 678-82.

[4] Clohisy, J.C., et al., *A systematic approach to the plain radiographic evaluation of the young adult hip.* J Bone Joint Surg Am, 2008. 90 Suppl 4: p. 47-66.

[5] Notzli, H.P., et al., *The contour of the femoral head-neck junction as a predictor for the risk of anterior impingement.* Journal of Bone & Joint Surgery - British Volume, 2002. 84(4): p. 556-60.

[6] De Pellegrin, M.P., W.G. Mackenzie, and H.T. Harcke, *Ultrasonographic evaluation of hip morphology in osteochondrodysplasias.* Journal of Pediatric Orthopedics, 2000. 20(5): p. 588-93.

[7] Beck, M., et al., *Hip morphology influences the pattern of damage to the acetabular cartilage: femoroacetabular impingement as a cause of early osteoarthritis of the hip.* Journal of Bone & Joint Surgery - British Volume, 2005. 87(7): p. 1012-8.

[8] McCarthy, J.C. and J.A. Lee, *Hip arthroscopy: indications, outcomes, and complications.* Instructional Course Lectures, 2006. 55: p. 301-8.

[9] Salvo, J.P., C.R. Troxell, and D.P. Duggan, *Incidence of venous thromboembolic disease following hip arthroscopy.* Orthopedics, 2010. 33(9): p. 664.

[10] Philippon, M., et al., *Femoroacetabular impingement in 45 professional athletes: associated pathologies and return to sport following arthroscopic decompression.* Knee Surg Sports Traumatol Arthrosc, 2007. 15(7): p. 908-14.

[11] Sampson, T.G., *Arthroscopic treatment of femoroacetabular impingement: a proposed technique with clinical experience.* Instr Course Lect, 2006. 55: p. 337-46.

[12] Byrd, J.W. and K.S. Jones, *Arthroscopic femoroplasty in the management of cam-type femoroacetabular impingement.* Clin Orthop Relat Res, 2009. 467(3): p. 739-46.

[13] Philippon, M.J., et al., *Outcomes following hip arthroscopy for femoroacetabular impingement with associated chondrolabral dysfunction: minimum two-year follow-up.* J Bone Joint Surg Br, 2009. 91(1): p. 16-23.

[14] Clohisy, J.C., et al., *Combined hip arthroscopy and limited open osteochondroplasty for anterior femoroacetabular impingement.* J Bone Joint Surg Am, 2010. 92(8): p. 1697-706.

[15] Pierannunzii, L. and M. d'Imporzano, *Treatment of femoroacetabular impingement: a modified resection osteoplasty technique through an anterior approach.* Orthopedics, 2007. 30(2): p. 96-102.

[16] Sink, E.L., et al., *Multicenter Study of Complications Following Surgical Dislocation of the Hip.* J Bone Joint Surg Am, 2011.

[17] Brooker, A.F., et al., *Ectopic ossification following total hip replacement. Incidence and a method of classification.* J Bone Joint Surg Am, 1973. 55(8): p. 1629-32.

[18] Murphy, S., et al., *Debridement of the adult hip for femoroacetabular impingement: indications and preliminary clinical results.* Clin Orthop Relat Res, 2004(429): p. 178-81.

[19] Peters, C.L. and J.A. Erickson, Treatment of femoro-acetabular impingement with surgical dislocation and debridement in young adults. J Bone Joint Surg Am, 2006. 88(8): p. 1735-41.

[20] Beaule, P.E., M.J. Le Duff, and E. Zaragoza, Quality of life following femoral head-neck osteochondroplasty for femoroacetabular impingement. J Bone Joint Surg Am, 2007. 89(4): p. 773-9.

[21] Espinosa, N., et al., Treatment of femoro-acetabular impingement: preliminary results of labral refixation. J Bone Joint Surg Am, 2006. 88(5): p. 925-35.

[22] Beck, M., et al., Anterior femoroacetabular impingement: part II. Midterm results of surgical treatment. Clin Orthop Relat Res, 2004(418): p. 67-73.

[23] Klaue, K., C.W. Durnin, and R. Ganz, The acetabular rim syndrome. A clinical presentation of dysplasia of the hip. Journal of Bone & Joint Surgery - British Volume, 1991. 73(3): p. 423-9.

[24] Murphy, S.B., R. Ganz, and M.E. Muller, The prognosis in untreated dysplasia of the hip. A study of radiographic factors that predict the outcome. Journal of Bone & Joint Surgery - American Volume, 1995. 77(7): p. 985-9.

[25] Schramm, M., et al., The Wagner spherical osteotomy of the acetabulum. Surgical technique. Journal of Bone & Joint Surgery - American Volume, 2004. 86-A Suppl 1: p. 73-80.

[26] Ganz, R., et al., A new periacetabular osteotomy for the treatment of hip dysplasias. Technique and preliminary results. Clin Orthop Relat Res, 1988(232): p. 26-36.

[27] Reynolds, D., J. Lucas, and K. Klaue, Retroversion of the acetabulum. A cause of hip pain. Journal of Bone & Joint Surgery - British Volume, 1999. 81(2): p. 281-8.

[28] Jamali, A.A., et al., Anteroposterior pelvic radiographs to assess acetabular retroversion: high validity of the "cross-over-sign". Journal of Orthopaedic Research, 2007. 25(6): p. 758-65.

[29] Matheney, T., et al., Intermediate to long-term results following the Bernese periacetabular osteotomy and predictors of clinical outcome. J Bone Joint Surg Am, 2009. 91(9): p. 2113-23.

[30] Garbuz, D.S., M.A. Awwad, and C.P. Duncan, Periacetabular osteotomy and total hip arthroplasty in patients older than 40 years. Journal of Arthroplasty, 2008. 23(7): p. 960-3.

[31] Matheney, T., et al., Intermediate to long-term results following the bernese periacetabular osteotomy and predictors of clinical outcome: surgical technique. J Bone Joint Surg Am, 2010. 92 Suppl 1 Pt 2: p. 115-29.

[32] Clohisy, J.C., et al., Periacetabular osteotomy: a systematic literature review. Clin Orthop Relat Res, 2009. 467(8): p. 2041-52.

[33] Davey, J.P. and R.F. Santore, Complications of periacetabular osteotomy. Clin Orthop Relat Res, 1999(363): p. 33-7.

[34] Ganz, R., et al., A new periacetabular osteotomy for the treatment of hip dysplasias. Technique and preliminary results. Clinical Orthopaedics & Related Research, 1988(232): p. 26-36.

[35] Trousdale, R.T., et al., Periacetabular and intertrochanteric osteotomy for the treatment of osteoarthrosis in dysplastic hips. J Bone Joint Surg Am, 1995. 77(1): p. 73-85.

[36] Peters, C.L., J.A. Erickson, and J.L. Hines, Early results of the Bernese periacetabular osteotomy: the learning curve at an academic medical center. J Bone Joint Surg Am, 2006. 88(9): p. 1920-6.

[37] Haverkamp, D. and R.K. Marti, Intertrochanteric osteotomy combined with acetabular shelfplasty in young patients with severe deformity of the femoral head and secondary osteoarthritis. A long-term follow-up study. J Bone Joint Surg Br, 2005. 87(1): p. 25-31.

[38] Chiari, K., *Medial displacement osteotomy of the pelvis*. Clin Orthop Relat Res, 1974(98): p. 55-71.

[39] Love, B.R., P.M. Stevens, and P.F. Williams, *A long-term review of shelf arthroplasty*. J Bone Joint Surg Br, 1980. 62(3): p. 321-5.

[40] Callaghan, J.J., R.A. Brand, and D.R. Pedersen, *Hip arthrodesis. A long-term follow-up*. Journal of Bone & Joint Surgery - American Volume, 1985. 67(9): p. 1328-35.

[41] Hamadouche, M., et al., Total hip arthroplasty for the treatment of ankylosed hips : a five to twenty-one-year follow-up study. J Bone Joint Surg Am, 2001. 83-A(7): p. 992-8.

[42] Joshi, A.B., et al., *Conversion of a fused hip to total hip arthroplasty*. J Bone Joint Surg Am, 2002. 84-A(8): p. 1335-41.

[43] Bittar, E.S. and W. Petty, *Girdlestone arthroplasty for infected total hip arthroplasty*. Clin Orthop Relat Res, 1982(170): p. 83-7.

4

Hip Fracture in the Elderly:
Partial or Total Arthroplasty?

Samo K. Fokter[1] and Nina Fokter[2]
[1]Celje General and Teaching Hospital
[2]Maribor University Clinical Centre
Slovenia

1. Introduction

The growing number of femoral neck fractures will have a large impact on health economics of developed countries in the coming decades. Great numbers of patients are already hospitalised yearly due to femoral neck fractures. These numbers are expected to augment importantly in the future years as the life expectancy and osteoporosis incidence increase in the ageing population. In the past, conservation of femoral head was supposed to be the ideal treatment for dislocated femoral neck fractures. However, conservation of femoral head with internal fixation has shown a high incidence of aseptic necrosis and non-union. Therefore, this treatment is now mostly applied to younger patients without osteoporosis and arthritis. In this chapter we review the topic of management of displaced femoral neck fractures in the elderly from a historical, surgical, and economical perspective. The emphasis is placed on the treatment rationale, surgical technique, and long-term clinical results. The authors' preferred choice of treatment of these sometimes difficult cases is also presented and illustrated.

2. Internal fixation or arthroplasty?

Therapeutic approaches for treatment of elderly patients with dislocated femoral neck fractures (Garden III-IV) include internal fixation of bone fragments, hemiarthroplasty or total hip arthroplasty (THA), and there is still no consensus about the optimal treatment. In a large multicentre prospective randomised study Rogmark et al. compared the results of internal fixation and hip arthroplasty in patients older than 70 years with a 2-year follow-up (Rogmark et al., 2002). They found 43% of treatment failures in the internal fixation group and only 6% of treatment failures in the arthroplasty group.

Bhandari et al. performed a meta-analysis of 14 prospective randomised studies comparing internal fixation with arthroplasty and discovered that 17% of patients could have been spared a revision surgery had they been treated with arthroplasty instead of internal fixation (Bhandari et al., 2003). Similar findings were described by Keating et al. in a study of patients older than 60 years with femoral neck fracture (Keating et al., 2006). At 2-year follow-up, 39% of the patients treated with internal fixation needed a secondary surgical procedure, whereas secondary surgery was required only in 5% of the patients treated with hemiarthroplasty and in 9% of the patients treated with THA. The complication rate can certainly be lowered by fast diagnostic procedures and a shorter time in bed waiting for the surgery. Internal fixation with femoral head preservation should be performed in the first 6 hours after the injury or only exceptionally in the first 24 hours. In older injuries hip arthroplasty should be performed (Sendtner et al., 2010). The bone healing potential is especially low in older patients (Figure 1).

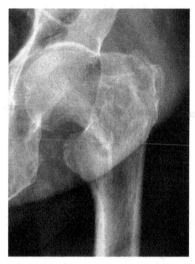

Fig. 1A. Proximal femoral fracture in a 74-year old female osteoporotic patient.

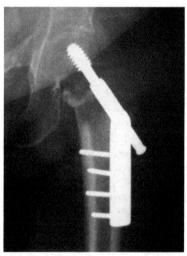

Fig. 1B. No signs of bony healing 6 months after open reduction and internal fixation with a dynamic hip screw (DHS) device. The patient is unable to walk.

In case we do not decide for preservation of the femoral head the remaining treatment options are unipolar hemiarthroplasty, bipolar hemiarthroplasty and THA.

3. Hemiarthroplasty

While hemiarthroplasty avoids the known risks of internal fixation, it brings other risks of its own: infection, stem loosening, dislocation, and groin pain as an effect of acetabular protrusion (Figure 2) or cartilage erosion (the so-called endoprosthetic arthritis).

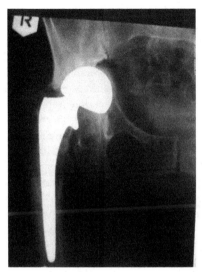

Fig. 2A. Acetabular fracture in a 64-year old patient 5 years after bipolar hemiarthroplasty for right femoral neck fracture.

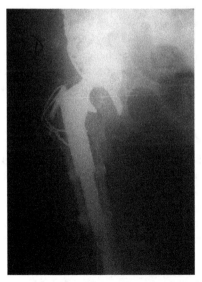

Fig. 2B. The same patient after revision total hip arthroplasty with insertion of a Bursch-Schneider acetabular supportive ring.

Unipolar hemiarthroplasty has been in use for more than half a century. The short-term results of this treatment are usually good, with rare infections and dislocations. However, the rates of mid- and long-term complications (5 to >20 years postoperatively) are high due to acetabular cartilage erosion. The cartilage defect causes pain and is the main reason for conversion to THA. Kofoed and Kofod found that as much as 55% of patients living alone needed conversion to THA two years after unipolar arthroplasty for femoral neck fracture (Kofoed & Kofod, 1983). The factors accelerating acetabular cartilage erosion are young age, high activity level and the length of follow-up (Macaulay et al., 2006).

The aim of introducing bipolar hemiarthroplasty in the 1970s was to prevent the development of endoprosthetic arthritis. Some motion is carried out among the components of the prosthesis, which theoretically diminishes acetabular wear. However, the functional importance of the prosthesis-prosthesis motion remains unclear. In a prospective randomised study of 115 patients over the age of 65 years with dislocated femoral neck fracture treated with either unipolar or bipolar hemiarthroplasty, Raija et al. found no statistical difference between the groups in quality of life and functional outcome at one year follow-up (Raija et al., 2003). Cornell et al. compared the results of treatment of 47 patients with an average age of 77 years. They noted better hip rotation and abduction and higher walking speed in the group treated with bipolar hemiarthroplasty compared to the group treated with unipolar hemiarthroplasty. On the other hand, they found no statistical difference in postoperative complication rates, lengths of hospitalisation and functional outcomes between the two groups (Cornell et al., 1998). Similar conclusions were reached by Parker and Gurusamy who compared the results of prospective randomised trials including a total of 857 patients (Parker & Gurusamy, 2004). The research showed an absence of significant differences between unipolar and bipolar hemiarthroplasty concerning hip dislocation, acetabular cartilage erosion, infection, reoperation rate and deep vein thrombosis at an average follow-up of 2 years.

Unipolar hemiarthroplasty is generally recommended for elderly, less active patients with a shorter life expectancy. These are the patients with the least benefit from the potential advantages of the more expensive bipolar hemiarthroplasty. Some authors advise against bipolar hemiarthroplasty in the elderly because of its higher price, long-term complications due to polyethylene wear, and higher rates of hip dislocations requiring an open reposition (Giliberty, 1983).

4. Total hip arthroplasty

In the past, THA was used in elderly patients with femoral neck fractures only in cases of coexisting acetabular disease. In 2004 Healy and Iorio proved that elderly patients treated with THA for displaced femoral neck fractures achieved a more independent living, a longer interval to reoperation or death, and better cost effectiveness than patients treated with internal fixation or hemiarthroplasty (Healy & Iorio, 2004).

Older studies have reported a higher incidence of hip dislocations after THA for femoral neck fractures compared to elective THA for acetabular cartilage disease. The reason for the higher dislocation rate was supposed to be the greater range of motion in patients with a fractured femoral neck. However, more recent studies have not confirmed the supposed differences concerning perioperative morbidity, functional outcome, and radiological signs of loosening (Abboud et al., 2004). Enocson et al. nevertheless recommended a careful choice of surgical approach in order to minimise the risk of dislocation (Enocson et al., 2009). In a prospective cohort study including 698 patients treated with THA for displaced femoral neck fracture or its complications, the least dislocations were noted in the anterolateral approach group (2%), while the dislocation rate in the posterolateral approach group was six times higher (13%). An additional reduction of dislocation risk in THA inserted via posterior approach can be achieved with the use of cemented dual articulation acetabular component (Tarasevicius et al., 2010).

Longer-term results of THA for femoral neck fracture were published by Lee et al. (Lee et al., 1998). They reported on treatment of 126 patients with an average age of 75 years and a 9-year follow-up. 10% of the patients had one or more postoperative dislocations, but 99% had mild or no pain and 69% reached their preoperative level of function or better. The study showed a higher complication rate in THA than is usual for hemiarthroplasty, but on the other hand revealed good clinical results and long-term prosthesis survival.

Total hip arthroplasty is a durable treatment option for femoral neck fractures in the elderly and gives a good functional outcome, but comes with the price of a higher complication rate, such as dislocation or postoperative delirium (Gallo et al., 2010). Surgical technique adapted to osteoporotic bone and careful implant selection regarding fixation influence the success of treatment for femoral neck fractures (Figure 3). The risk of dislocation depends on the surgical approach, the reconstruction of hip biomechanics, the head size and offset, the quality of capsular closure, and the experience of the surgeon (Ames et al., 2010; Leighton et al., 2007; Rutz et al., 2010).

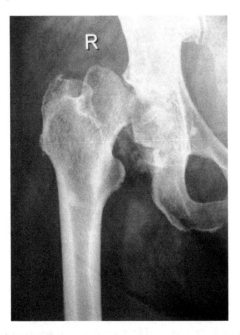

Fig. 3A. Subcapital fracture in a 71-year old female patient with osteoporosis.

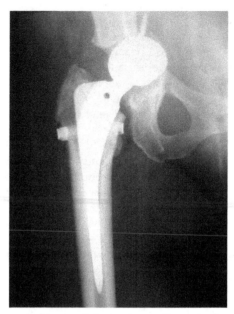

Fig. 3B. Acetabular fracture and intrapelvic cup (press-fit type) migration noted 6 weeks after primary uncemented THA in the same patient. Note that intraoperative femoral shaft fracture also occurred and was treated with a cerclage belt.

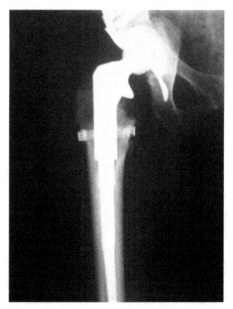

Fig. 3C. The same patient after revision THA with modular femoral stem and a Bursch-Schneider acetabular supportive ring.

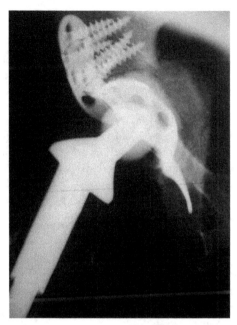

Fig. 3D. The same patient after revision THA on lateral radiograph. Note massive autologous bone grafts under the Bursch-Schneider ring.

5. Cemented or cementless hip arthroplasty?

There is still a lively ongoing debate in the orthopaedic community as to which method of fixation of the implant is superior to the other. Although the development of total hip replacement began with cementless THA in the late fifties, cemented THA has been more popular after Charnley's systematic promotion of low friction arthroplasty, which included fixation with bone cement (Charnley, 1961). Nevertheless, cementless THA rapidly gained acceptance during the 1980s when materials that allowed bone ingrowth became available. A meta-analysis comparing the survival rate of cemented and cementless THA reported that cemented THA was slightly superior (Morsched et al., 2007). However, the difference between the groups was no longer significant when revision surgery of the cup or the stem was regarded as treatment failure. At present, it is not possible to ascertain the superiority of any of the two options. In the authors' institutions, cemented type of fixation is used in the majority of fracture cases.

Figved et al. recently raised the question whether a specific type of fixation should be used for the treatment of displaced femoral neck fractures (Figved et al., 2009). In the randomized, controlled trial in patients 70 years and older comparing a cemented implant with hydroxyapatite-coated uncemented implant, both with a bipolar head, the mean Harris hip score showed equivalence between the groups after 3 months and 12 months. The complication and mortality rates were similar in both groups. However, the duration of surgery was 12.4 minutes shorter and the mean intraoperative blood loss was 89 mL less in the cementless group.

6. Hemiarthroplasty or total hip arthroplasty?

Rogmark et al. tried to evaluate which patients to treat with THA and which with hemiarthroplasty in the course of surgical treatment of femoral neck fractures (Rogmark et al., 2002). In the multicentre prospective randomised trial comparing internal fixation to arthroplasty, they divided the arthroplasty group to hemiarthroplasty and THA according to the scoring system for patients with femoral neck fracture (Table 1). Patients with a score of 15 or more were treated with THA and the others with hemiarthroplasty. The scoring system favoured THA in younger (age 70-80 years), alert patients who were capable of independent walking before the injury. The authors noted no significant difference between the THA and hemiarthroplasty groups. The overall dislocation rate was 8%. They concluded that the good functional outcome and the relatively low incidence of dislocations proved the value of their scoring system for choosing the appropriate patients for each treatment option.

Patient Variables	Points*
Age	
70 to 80 years	5
> 80 years	2
Habitat	
Own home	5
Sheltered home	2
Walking aids	
One cane or none	5
Canes, walking frame	2
Mental status	
Alert	5
Slight confusion	2

*A total score ≥15 points indicates treatment required with total hip arthroplasty.

Table 1. Rogmark preoperative scoring system for patients with femoral neck fractures (Rogmark et al., 2002).

Hopley et al. recently published a systematic review comparing THA with hemiarthroplasty considering reoperation rates, mortality, complications, functional outcome and quality of life (Hopley et al., 2010). They identified 3821 references, inspected 202 papers and included 15 papers with a total of 1890 patients. The meta-analysis showed that THA carried a lower risk of reoperation than hemiarthroplasty. THA also showed better ratings in the Harris hip score than hemiarthroplasty. However, the rates of dislocation (relative risk 1.48; 95% confidence interval 0.89 to 2.46) and general complications (relative risk 1.14, 95% confidence interval 0.87 to 1.48) were slightly higher for THA.

Arthroplasty is thus indicated in most patients over the age of 65 years with femoral neck fractures. Hemiarthroplasty is indicated in institutionalised patients and patients with comorbidities who are not expected to live longer than 6 or 7 years. Studies show a high reoperation rate in patients living longer than 6 to 7 years after hemiarthroplasty. THA is indicated in active patients with little or no comorbidities as it represents the most successful treatment in terms of pain relief and is also cost effective (Kyle, 2010). Recent advances in the materials and technology of THA components allowing the use of larger femoral heads, as well as better surgical techniques have made THA safer and less prone to dislocation and other mechanical complications. Economical analyses demonstrate that due to the costs of complications THA is more cost effective than internal fixation or hemiarthroplasty in patients surviving 2 years or longer after their initial femoral neck fracture. An increasing number of authors therefore believe that THA should be granted a larger role in the treatment of displaced femoral neck fractures than it has had in the past (Schmidt et al., 2009).

7. Cost

We live in a time of global recession and information about the cost of treatment is unfortunately not unimportant. Iorio et al. calculated the costs of treatment of femoral neck fractures in the elderly during a 2-year postoperative period (Iorio et al., 2001). Surgical treatment methods included reduction with internal fixation, unipolar hemiarthroplasty, bipolar hemiarthroplasty, and THA. The analysis included the costs of hospitalisation, rehabilitation, and probability-adjusted costs of revision. The calculated total cost of cemented THA was 20,670 US dollars, hybrid THA 21,066 US dollars, bipolar hemiarthroplasty 22,043 US dollars, unipolar hemiarthroplasty 21,597 US dollars, and internal fixation 24,606 US dollars. The authors concluded that taking into account complication rates, mortality, revision surgeries and functional outcome, THA is the most cost effective treatment option for femoral neck fractures in the elderly.

The current costs of treatment for femoral neck fractures in the elderly in Northern Europe have been analysed by Frihagen et al. (Frihagen et al., 2010). They randomised 222 patients with an average age of 83 years to internal fixation or hemiarthroplasty. The patients were followed for 2 years. The analysis included costs of hospitalisation, rehabilitation, community-based care, and nursing home use. Primary hospital treatment was less expensive in the group treated with internal fixation (9,044 euros) than in the hemiarthroplasty group (11,887 euros). The relation changed when they included all hospital costs (rehabilitation, revision surgeries, formal and informal contact with the hospital): 21,709 euros for internal fixation and 19,976 euros for hemiarthroplasty. When all costs of the 2-year treatment were included (with community-based care and nursing home), internal fixation was much more expensive (47,186 euros) than hemiarthroplasty (38,615 euros).

8. Summary

Strong evidence exists in favour of primary arthroplasty over internal fixation for displaced femoral neck fractures in the elderly. Hemiarthroplasty is indicated for institutionalised patients, and patients with comorbidities who are not expected to live longer than a few years. THA is definitely indicated for patients with concurrent degenerative or rheumatic arthritis. Besides, evidence is accumulating that THA may be more effective than hemiarthroplasty in terms of pain relief and functional outcome in younger, more active patients with intact acetabulum and longer life expectancy. Regarding costs to the society, hemiarthroplasty is more favourable than internal fixation on the short term, and THA is more favourable than hemiarthroplasty on the medium term. Considering the growing life expectancy, primary THA should be chosen more often for the treatment of displaced femoral neck fractures even in the elderly.

9. References

Abboud, J. A., Patel, R. V., Booth Jr, R. E. & Nasarian, D. G. (2004). Outcomes of total hip arthroplasty are similar for patients with displaced femoral neck fractures and osteoarthritis. *Clinical Orthopaedics and Related Research*, Vol.421, No.4, (April 2004), pp. 151-154

Ames, J. B., Lurie, J. D., Tomek, I. M., Zhou, W. & Koval, K. J. (2010) Does surgeon volume for total hip arthroplasty affect outcomes after hemiarthroplasty for femoral neck fracture? *The American Journal of Orthopedics (Belle Mead)*, Vol.39, No.8, (August 2010), pp. E84-89

Bhandari, M., Devereaux, P. J., Swiontkowski, M. F., Tornetta 3rd, P., Obremskey, W., Koval, K. J., Nork, S., Sprague, S., Schemitsch, E. H. & Guyatt, G. H. (2003) Internal fixation compared with arthroplasty for displaced fractures of the femoral neck: A meta-analysis. *Journal of Bone and Joint Surgery, American Volume*, Vol.85, No.9, (September 2003), pp. 1673-1681

Charnley, J. (1961) Arthroplasty of the hip: A new operation. *Lancet*, Vol.277, No.7187, (May 1961), pp. 1129-1132

Cornell, C. N., Levine, D., O'Doherty, J. & Lyden, J. (1998) Unipolar versus bipolar hemiarthroplasty for the treatment of femoral neck fractures in the elderly. *Clinical Orthopaedics and Related Research*, Vol.348, No.3, (March 1998), pp. 67-71

Enocson, A., Hedbeck, C. J., Tidermark, J., Pettersson, H., Ponzer, S. & Lapidus, L. J. (2009) Dislocation of total hip replacement in patients with fractures of the femoral neck: A prospective cohort study of 713 consecutive hips. *Acta Ortopaedica*, Vol.80, No.2, (April 2009), pp. 184-189, ISSN 1745-3674

Figved, W., Opland, V., Frihagen, F., Jervidalo, T., Madsen, J. E. & Nordsletten, L. (2009) Cemented versus uncemented hemiarthroplasty for displaced femoral neck fractures. *Clinical Orthopaedics and Related Research*, Vol.467, No.9, (September 2009), pp. 2426-2435

Frihagen, F., Waaler, G. M., Madsen, J. E., Nordsletten, L., Aspaas, S. & Aas, E. (2010) The cost of hemiarthroplasty to that of internal fixation for femoral neck fractures. *Acta Orthopaedica*, Vol.81, No.4, (August 2010), pp. 446-452

Gallo, J., Cechova, I. & Zapletalova, J. (2010) Early complications associated with total hip arthroplasty due to femoral neck fracture. *Acta Chirurgiae Orthopaedicae et Traumatologiae Cechoslovaca*, Vol.77, No.5, (October 2010), pp. 389-394

Giliberty, R. P. (1983) Hemiarthroplasty of the hip using low-friction bipolar endoprosthesis. *Clinical Orthopaedics and Related Research*, Vol.175, No.5, (May 1983), pp. 86-92

Healy, W. L. & Iorio, R. (2004) Total hip arthroplasty: Optimal treatment for displaced femoral neck fractures in elderly patients. *Clinical Orthopaedics and Related Research*, Vol.429, No.12, (December 2004), pp. 43-48

Hopley, C., Stengel, D., Ekkernkamp, A. & Wich, M. (2010) Primary total hip arthroplasty versus hemiarthroplasty for displaced intracapsular hip fractures in older patients: Systematic review. *British Medical Journal*, No.340, (June 2010), c2332

Iorio, R., Healy, W. L., Lemos, D. W., Appleby, D., Luzzhesi, C. A. & Saleh, K. J. (2001) Displaced femoral neck fractures in the elderly: Outcomes and cost effectiveness. *Clinical Orthopaedics and Related Research*, Vol.383, No.2, (February 2001), pp. 229-242

Keating, J. F., Grant, A., Masson, M., Scott, N. W. & Forbes, J. F. (2006) Randomized comparison of reduction and fixation, bipolar hemiarthroplasty, and total hip arthroplasty: Treatment of displaced intracapsular hip fractures in healthy older patients. *Journal of Bone and Joint Surgery, American Volume*, Vol.88, No.2, (February 2006), pp. 249-60

Kofoed, H. & Kofod, J. (1983) Moore prosthesis in the treatment of fresh femoral neck fractures: A critical review with special attention to secondary acetabular degeneration. *Injury*, Vol.14, No.6, (May 1983), pp. 531-540

Kyle, R. F. (2010) Subcapital fractures: In the bucket or on top of the neck? *Orthopedics*, Vol.33, No.9, (September 2010), p.644

Lee, B. P., Berry, D. J., Harmsen, W. S. & Sim, F. H. (1998) Total hip arthroplasty for the treatment of an acute fracture of the femoral neck: Long-term results. *Journal of Bone and Joint Surgery, American Volume*, Vol.80, No.1, (January 1998), pp. 70-75

Leighton, R. K., Schmidt, A. H., Collier, P. & Trask, K. (2007) Advances in the treatment of intracapsular hip fractures in the elderly. *Injury*, Vol.38, No.S3, (September 2007), pp.S24-S34

Macaulay, W., Pagnotto, M. R., Iorio, R., Mont, M. A. & Saleh, K. J. (2006) Displaced femoral neck fractures in the elderly: hemiarthroplasty versus total hip arthroplasty. *Journal of the American Academy of Orthopaedic Surgeons*, Vol.14, No.5, (May 2006), pp. 287-293

Morsched, S., Bozic, K. J., Ries, M. D., Malchau, H. & Colford Jr., J. M. (2007) Comparison of cemented and uncemented fixation in total hip replacement: a meta-analysis. *Acta Orthopaedica*, Vol.78, No.3, (June 2007), pp. 315-326

Parker, M. J. & Gurusamy, K. (2004) Arthroplasties (with and without bone cement) for proximal femoral fractures in adults. *Cochrane Database of Systematic Reviews*, Vol.2, CD001706

Raia, F. J., Chapman, C. B., Herrera, M., Schweppe, M. W., Michelsen, C. B. & Rosenwasser, M. P. (2003) Unipolar or bipolar hemiarthroplasty for femoral neck fractures in the elderly? *Clinical Orthopaedics and Related Research*, Vol.414, No.9, (September 2003), pp. 259-265

Rogmark, C., Carlsson, A., Johnell, O. & Sernbo, I. (2002) A prospective randomised trial of internal fixation versus arthroplasty for displaced fractures of the neck of the femur: Functional outcomes for 450 patients at two years. *Journal of Bone and Joint Surgery, British Volume*, Vol.84, No.2, (March 2002), pp. 183-188

Rutz, E., Leumann, A., Rutz, D., Schaefer, D. & Walderrabano, W. (2010) Total hip arthroplasty for fractures of the proximal femur in older patients. *Hip International*, Vol.20, No.2, (April-June 2010), pp. 215-220

Schmidt, A. H., Leighton, R., Parvizi, J., Sems, A. & Berry, D. J. (2009) Optimal arthroplasty for femoral neck fractures: Is total hip arthroplasty the answer? *Journal of Orthopaedic Trauma*, Vol.23, No.6, (July 2009), pp. 428-433

Sendtner, E., Renkawitz, T., Kramny, P., Wenzl, M. & Grifka, J. (2010) Fractured neck of femur – internal fixation versus arthroplasty. *Deutsches Aerzteblatt International,* Vol.107, No.23, (June 2010), pp.401-407

Tarasevicius, S., Busevicius, M., Robertson, O. & Wingstrand, H. (2010) Dual mobility cup reduces dislocation rate after arthroplasty for femoral neck fracture. *BMC Musculoskeletal Disorders,* Vol.6, No.11, (August 2010), pp. 175-178

5

Minimally Invasive Total Hip Arthroplasty

Mel S. Lee

College of Medicine, Chang Gung University,
Department of Orthopedic Surgery, Chang Gung Memorial Hospital at Linkou
Taiwan

1. Introduction

Total hip arthroplasty (THA) is one of the most reliable procedures that can provide short-term high clinical success rates and long-term durable outcome. The surgery has been developed for more than 40 years and most of the clinical practices are standardized for the patient care. In the past, THA had been done by making a wound about 25 cm in length. Many surgeons believed that big wounds should be the standard approach for THA because the surgery is a big surgery and could only be reliably done with big wounds. In recent 10 years, this concept of "big surgery-big wound" has been challenged in many fields of surgery. Taking the arthroscopic ligament reconstruction surgery or laparoscopic cholecystectomy surgery as the examples, many surgical procedures can now be safely and adequately performed by the minimally invasive (MIS) approaches. Although impossibly be done by an arthroscopy, the surgical approaches for THA have been adopting the concept of MIS and modified by many surgeons. However, the definition of a MIS-THA is not as straightforward as the words meanings. Based on the incision length, it is generally agreed upon that an incision less than 10 cm can be defined as MIS-THA. However the MIS can also be interpreted as less soft tissue trauma or less bone tissue trauma when doing the THA. The incision wound length then is not necessarily equal to the extent of tissue injury during the procedure. To date, the MIS-THA can be divided into two categories. One decreases the wound and muscle cutting and emphasizes the tissue repair through either a lateral or a posterior route. [1-4] The other spares muscle sectioning during the procedure through one [5,6], two [1,7-11], or multiple [12] incisions. The abridged incision methods minimize the incision length and can be extensile if difficulties are encountered during THA. The muscle sparing methods use tissue intervals for surgery but could be difficult if complications happened intraoperatively. In the literature, the complication rates are significantly higher in inexperienced, low-volume surgeons in the "learning curve" period for the muscle sparing techniques. [13] THA, however, is a reliable procedure and its clinical results should not be compromised by the surgical approaches. For those surgeons who start to learn the procedure, standard surgical approach with bigger wounds is strongly recommended.
In the learning curve period of the MIS-THA, the incision should start from a standard length and then gradually reduces its size as the experiences accumulated. To master the MIS-THA surgical techniques, surgeons also need to familiar with the anatomy and different surgical approaches for THA. [14]

2. Surgical approaches for total hip arthroplasty

For the surgical approaches, THA can be done by different routes. Each approach has its potential advantages and limitations. Followings are the commonly used approaches for THA.

2.1 The transtrochanteric approach

The transtrochanteric approach osteotomizes the greater trochanter and retracts it along with the gluteal medius and minimus anteriorly to facilitate exposure. It is nowadays seldom performed on primary cases and is performed selectively on revision cases, secondary reconstruction after hip fractures, and for distal transfer of the greater trochanter. The transtrochanteric approach is originally done at the level between the insertion of hip abductors and the origin of the vastus lateralis. It is however associated with complications such as nonunion or proximal migration of the greater trochanter that often result in weakness of the abductors with marked limping gait or even instability of the THA. To avoid proximal migration of the greater trochanter and enhance the union rates, both the insertion of gluteal muscles and the origin of the vastus lateralis can be preserved on the greater trochanter as a whole construct and be slide anteriorly during the procedure. The trochanteric slide or flip approach prevents untoward proximal migration of the greater trochanter and enhances the fixation stability of the trochanter. [15] The trochanteric slide technique can be further modified by extending the osteotomy to the lateral cortex of the proximal femur to facilitate implant or cement removal in complex cases. [16]

2.2 The transgluteal approach (direct lateral)

The transgluteal approach splits the gluteal medius along its muscle fibers and cut about one third or half of the gluteal medius from its musculotendinous insertion on the trochanter. (**Figure 1**) The muscle is retracted ventrally and the underlying gluteal minimus

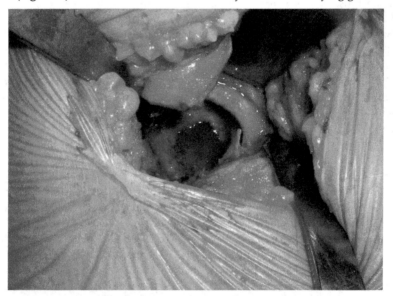

Fig. 1. The direct lateral approach detaches 1/3 of the gluteal medius from the greater trochanter to facilitate anterior dislocation of the hip joint.

and the joint capsule are then incised in a T-manner to facilitate anterior dislocation of the hip. In standard lateral approach of Hardinge [17], part of the vastus muscle can be incised to help the exposure. In modified method, the origins of the vastus muscle can be spared to decrease the tissue trauma. Possible risks of the approach involve an injury to the muscular braches of the superior gluteal nerve or direct injury to the muscle fibers by compression or retraction during surgery. This will result in damage to the gluteal muscles or muscular insufficiency and is associated with higher chance of Trendelenburg sign **(Figure 2)** postoperatively. [18]

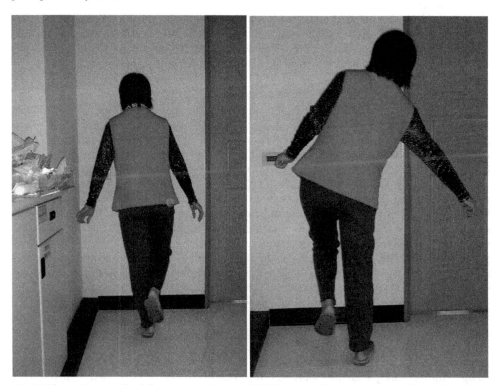

Fig. 2. The patient with abductors weakness. (A) When standing on the sound leg, the pelvis can be kept level and will not drop. (B) When standing on the affected leg, patient will compensatory list to the affected side to avoid pelvis dropping. (Duchenne sign)

2.3 The posterolateral approach

The posterolateral approach is probably the most popular surgical approach for THA for many orthopedic surgeons. Skin incision is made along the posterior border of the proximal femur centered on the top of the greater trochanter. The muscle part of the gluteal maximus is split along its fibers. The short external rotators and the posterior joint capsule are detached from the posterior border of the femur. The hip is dislocated posteriorly by internally rotation, flexion, and adduction. Cares should be taken to identify and protect the sciatic nerve during the procedure. After the THA, a secure and tight repair of the posterior capsule should be performed to decrease the dislocation rates. [3,4]

2.4 The anterolateral approach

Between the anatomical interval of the gluteal medius and tensor fascia latae superficially, the so-called Watson-Jones interval, the anterior hip joint capsule can be exposed by retracting the rectus femoris medially and the gluteal muscles laterally. During the exposure of the anterior femoral neck, the assistant can gradually rotate the leg in externally rotated position. Usually the neck should be cut in place because the complete anterior dislocation of the hip is difficult. The acetabulum is exposed by placing two retractors, one on the front to protect the rectus femoris and one on the back to push the femur posteriorly. The femur is exposed by placing the limb in hyperextension, adduction, and 90° external rotation. One retractor is placed behind the greater trochanter to protect the gluteus medius. One retractor is placed below the proximal medial neck to leverage the proximal femur for canal preparation. [5] Because only the fasica layers were split without detaching muscles from the hip, special retractors are often needed to facilitate exposure and dislocation of the hip.

2.5 The anterior approach

The direct anterior approach is usually performed with the patient in the supine position. [6] Dissection is in the Smith-Peterson interval between the fascia of the Sartorius muscle and the fascia of the tensor fascia lata muscle. The skin incision begins from a point distal to the anterior superior iliac spine and extends obliquely in the direction of the tensor fascia lata. By blunt dissection, the Sartorius muscle can be retracted medially and the muscle belly of the fascia lata can be retracted laterally. At this point, the underlying fascia between the rectus femoris and the inferior fasica layer of the tensor fascia lata can be exposed. In this layer, the ascending branches of the lateral femoral circumflex vessels can be identified and ligated. A Cobra retractor is put around the anterior inferior femoral neck above the capsule to elevate the reflected head of rectus femoris. Another Hohmann retractor is put around the posterior femoral neck and the posterior acetabulum to retract the gluteal muscles behind. Sometimes part of the reflected head of the rectus femoris need to be released to help the exposure. The anterior hip capsule can then be incised or excised. The retractors can then be put intra-articularly while cutting the femoral neck. For the aceabular preparation, visualization of the bony landmarks can be done by putting a Hohmann retractor under the posterior rim of acetabulum to push the proximal femur posteriorly and by another retractor on the medial wall of the acetabulum above the pubic bone. For femoral preparation, the leg needs to be positioned in hyperextension, adduction and external rotation. The posterior medial capsule along with the short external rotator muscles are released in a stepwise manner. The leg is put in the "figure of 4" position and a blunt Cobra retractor can be put behind the greater trochanter to gradually elevate the proximal femur.

2.6 The combined approach

By combining the above surgical routes, THA can also be done by the double incision methods [1,7-11] or the triple incision method [12]. The double incision method is a modified method of the direct anterior approach by Berger and Mears. [14] Patient is put in the supine position and the hip joint is approached via the Smith-Peterson interval. [7,8] The anterior skin incision is made along the long axis of the femoral neck. The fascia and muscle over the hip joint are split without cutting into their attachment. Two Hohmann retractors, one medial and one lateral to the femoral neck, are used to retract the gluteal medius laterally and the rectus femoris medially. The femoral neck needs to be cut in situ because dislocation of the hip joint is almost impossible by such a limited dissection. Usually the femoral neck needs to be doubly cut at the head-neck junction and at the standard neck cut level. After removing the bone block of the femoral neck, a space is created for the ease of femoral head retrieval. The acetabulum is prepared as the standard direct anterior approach. Another incision is made posterior to the greater trochanter. The fascia and muscles of the gluteal maximus are split in line with its muscle fibers. Similar to the technique of femoral intramedullary nailing, the femoral canal is prepared by sequential enlargement with reamers. Under the fluoroscopic guidance, both the acetabular and the femoral component can be implanted in predetermined position.

We and others have modified the two-incision technique by putting the patient in the lateral decubitus position [9-11]. The anterior skin incision is made perpendicular to the long axis of the femoral neck about 3 to 4 finger-breadth distal to the ilioinguinal line. **(Figure 3)** The hip joint is approached through the Smith-Peterson interval. Double neck cutting to the hip joint is also needed. While the anterior skin incision is made along the intertrochanteric line, the greater trochanter and the proximal femur can be visualized more easily by gentle retraction of the gluteus medius and tensor fascia lata. By this modification, the process of femoral canal preparation can be safely done under direct vision without the help of the fluoroscopic monitoring. [9-11,19]

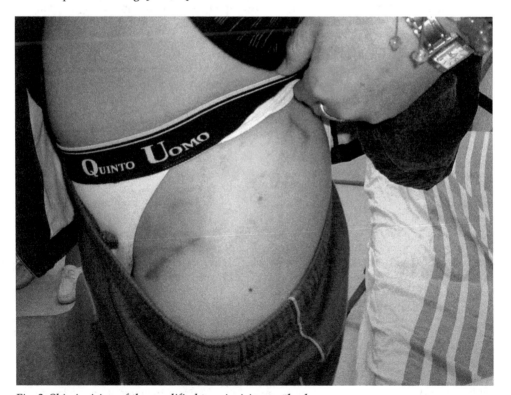

Fig. 3. Skin incision of the modified two-incision method.

The triple incision method is similar to the double incision method. It can be done with the patient in the supine or in the lateral decubitus position. Basically the incisions for the acetabulum and the femur exposure are not different from the original 2-incision method and the tissue intervals used for surgery are the same. The third incision is only needed in some heavy muscular or obese cases whereas the appropriate handling of the surgical instruments to the desirable position cannot be done. [12]

2.7 The omega approach

The approach is a lateral approach to the hip joint with the patient in the supine or lateral position. [20] Skin incision is centered over the greater trochanter. The fascia lata and gluteus maximus are split in the line of the skin incision. An aponeurotic flap including the gluteus medius and the vastus lateralis is elevated subperiosteally. The dissection starts proximally in the plane between the tendons of gluteus medius and piriformis. The attachments of gluteus medius and gluteus minimus from the greater trochanter are mobilized by sharp dissection. The dissection continues distally to involve the anterior border of the vastus lateralis as a single continuous strip of tissue. The shape of the incision resembles the Greek letter omega. Care should be taken to create the "osteoaponeurotic" flap as a whole construct. The entire muscle flap of gluteus medius, minimus, and vastus lateralis is mobilized off the anterior capsule of the hip. The hip capsule is incised in a T-shape manner. Subsequent repair of the osteoaponeurotic flap can be augmented by interrupted non-absorbable sutures by passing the sutures through holes drilled in the bone.

2.8 Patient positioning and special operation table

MIS-THA can be done with the patient in the supine or lateral position depending on the surgeon's preference. As a general rule, if the THA is performed from the anterior route, a supine position will be more intuitive. If the THA is performed from the lateral or posterolateral route, a lateral position should be easier for the surgeon. The patient positioning is important in performing the THA because the implant positions are often determined intraoperatively with the reference to the patient's position, bony anatomy, and the environmental setting. In MIS-THA, it is even more important because the bony anatomy and landmarks are sometimes less visualized. The proper patient positioning is also necessary during the THA because the operated leg needs to be manipulated in different directions and positions to facilitate hip dislocation, bone preparation, and check for the leg length equality.

In the supine position, a sandbag or an inflatable pillow can be put beneath the buttock to help the hyperextension of the hip. The foot-piece of the operative table on the operated side can be lowered and the leg can be put in a "figure of 4" position in hyperextension, adduction, and external rotation. The proximal femur then can be more easily accessed from the anterior wound. [21]

In the lateral position, the positions and directions of the operated leg depend on the surgical approaches for the femur preparation. With the posterolateral approach, the leg needs to be adducted, internally rotated, and flexed. With the transgluteal approach or omega approach, the leg needs to be adducted, externally rotated, and flexed. Both the posterolateral and the transgluteal approach can be done on a standard operation table. An operation table with the foot-piece that can be removed or lowered is required for the anterolateral (Watson-Jones) approach because during the femur preparation the leg needs to be adducted, externally rotated, and hyper-extended. (Figure 4) If the operation table is not available, the patient needs to be put toward the side of the table to facilitate the hip extension postion.

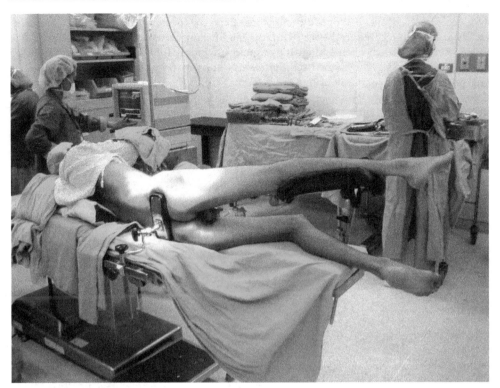

Fig. 4. The special operation table for modified Watson-Jones approach.

Matta et al. has described a unique method of THA using direct anterior approach to the hip. [22] The patient is put on a fracture table that the leg can be pulled by traction in extension and external rotation position. Fluoroscopy can be used during the procedure to control the leg length. However the technique needs a well organized surgical team to adjust the traction and fluoroscopy. Some rare complications such as the ankle fracture or calcaneal fracture have been reported.

2.9 MIS-THA

For many years, THA through a reduced wound has been performed in patients on a selective base by many surgeons. However in the past decade, the issue about MIS-THA has provoked great attention and controversy among the society and the publicity. The two-incision technique was publicized by Berger et al. in the Rush-Presbyterian University Hospital. [7,8] In the following years, many studies including prospective randomized trial, large cohort study, case control study, clinical series, and expert opinions about a variety of MIS-THA are reported. As described previously, the MIS-THA can be divided into two categories. The first is the abridged incision MIS-THA and the second is the muscle-sparing MIS-THA.

2.10 Abridged incision MIS-THA

Because the major difference between the abridged incision techniques and the conventional techniques is the length of incision, the abridged incision techniques are now more popular and acceptable to the orthopaedic surgeons than the muscle-sparing techniques. The abridged incision techniques basically are the modification of the conventional approaches by reducing the skin incision and creating a mobile window for surgical field visualization. Special instruments are designed for the ease of surgery **(Figure 5)** For the transgluteal approach to the hip joint, about one third to one half of the musculotendinous portion of gluteus medius and minimus are detached from the greater trochanter to facilitate anterior dislocation of the hip joint. Care should be taken not to damage the superior gluteal nerve by overstretching the muscle fibers. For the posterlateral MIS approach to the hip joint, the piriformis tendon or part of the quadratus femoris tendon can be preserved. The hip is dislocated posteriorly by internal rotation, adduction, and flexion. Emphasis has also been on the secure repair of the posterior capsule and the short external rotators after prosthesis implantation. By this modification, this approach proves to be a reliable and safe procedure and the dislocation rates are significantly decreased. [3,4]

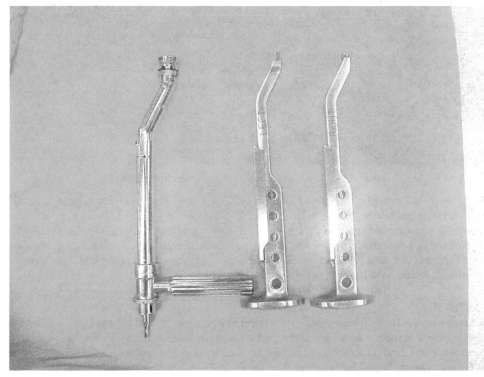

Fig. 5. Dog-legged instruments can be used to avoid skin and soft tissue impingement during MIS surgery.

2.11 Muscle-sparing MIS-THA

The muscle-sparing MIS-THA uses tissue intervals and avoids muscle sectioning for prosthesis implantation. Single-incision or multi-incision muscle-sparing MIS techniques have been described in the literatures. The single-incision techniques include the anterolateral (modified Watson-Jones) approach [5] and the direct anterior approach (Smith-

Peterson) [6,21,22]. The multiple-incision techniques include the two-incision approach [7-11] or the three-incision approach [12]. Although the muscle sparing MIS-THA techniques are also the modification of the classic anterior or anterolateral approach to the hip joint, these techniques are greatly different from the classic ones in terms of the skin incision and tissue dissection. Because the muscles around the hip joint are not cut or detached, dislocation of the hip for the ease of surgical exposure is difficult. Usually a double cut to the femoral neck is needed with one cut over the head-neck junction and the other cut at the desired position above the lesser trochanter.

In MIS direct anterior approach, both acetabular cup and femoral stem can be implanted in a single incision with the patients in the supine position. The single-incision techniques use the Smith-Peterson interval and can be facilitated by using a fracture table or by lowering the leg to hyperextend the hips. [6,21,22]

In the multi-incision techniques, the acetabular cup and femoral stem are separately implanted through different incisions depending on the musculatures and sizes of the patients. Patients can also be placed in supine or lateral position. Intraoperative fluoroscopy is usually advised because direct visualization of the femur during stem implantation is difficult. Under the fluoroscopic guidance, the procedure is very similar to the closed femoral intramedullary nailing technique. [7,8] However by modifying the direction of the skin incisions and position of the patients, the procedure could be done without intraoperative fluoroscopy because direct visualization of the proximal femur is possible. [1,9,10]

The muscle-sparing techniques are less popular than the abridged incision or the conventional techniques. The techniques are challenging and need a steeper learning curve because the surgical anatomy and surgical landmarks are less apprehensible among most surgeons and their surgical team members as well. Special instruments, operation table, or additional training are highly demanded to facilitate and to safe-guard the procedures.

2.12 Clinical results of the MIS-THA

The increasing popularity of MIS-THA has led to some debates regarding to the safety and clinical results for the "new technologies". Although a decade has been passed, the follow-up length is still inadequate and good quality randomized control studies are not enough to make a conclusion.

For the evaluation of abridged incision posterior approach, Ogonda had performed a randomized control trial by comparing the standard approach with the MIS-THA approach among different groups of surgeons. Ogonda et al. found the MIS-THA using mini-posterior approach was safe and reliable but provided no extra-benefit as compared to the standard posterior approach in terms of the functional outcomes and the ambulatory ability. [23,24] Kim reported on 60 simultaneous bilateral THA in 30 patients, with each patients serving as his or her own control. [25] The only difference between the MIS-THA and the standard THA was less blood loss in the MIS group. Dorr et al. had combined the imageless navigation system with the mini-posterior MIS-THA technique. They found the MIS-THA using the mini-posterior approach had shortened hospital stays, earlier mobility, less pain, and higher satisfaction in the early postoperative period. [3] The higher satisfaction among the patients with the MIS-THA is associated with the successful implementation of patient education and rehabilitation program. In the high motivated patients, the psychologic expectation and the physical recovery are more realistic. [26]

The muscle-sparing approaches include the direct anterior, the two- , or the three-incision techniques. Theoretically the muscle sparing techniques should have more rapid functional recovery because the muscles around the hip joint are not violated. As a matter of fact, the muscle sparing techniques are more difficult than the conventional or the abridged incision techniques. Pagnano et al. reported that the muscle-sparing two-incision technique had modest outcomes and substantial complications. [27] By using cadaver studies, they also found evidences of more muscles damage with the two-incision technique than the mini-posterior technique. [28] Others had reported some unusual catastrophic complications and heterotopic ossification by using the muscle-sparing technique. [29,30] As a contrast, high satisfaction and rapid recovery were consistently found in patients treated by experienced surgeons. [7,8,31] Duwelius et al. had compared the two-incision technique with the posterior MIS technique by using historical match-pair control cases and found that the mini-posterior technique had less blood loss and shorter operation time and the two-incision technique had better functional recovery and shorter hospital stays. [31] We had modified the two-incision technique by setting the patient in the lateral position and changed the orientation of the skin incision to facilitate the surgical exposure of the proximal femur. When compared with the standard transgluteal approach, the modified two-incision technique was proven to be safe and had comparable hospital courses and operative results. [1] Using dynamometer to check the muscular torques preoperatively and postoperatively, it was reported that the muscular recovery of the hip flexors were earlier in the postoperative period than the hip extensors by using the modified two-incision technique. [10]

The single-incision muscle-sparing MIS-THA are less reported in the literature except those from the technique developers. [5,6,21,22] Laffosse et al. had compared the anterolateral mini-invasive technique with the posterior mini-invasive approach and reported that both techniques had comparable surgical results and similar implant positioning. [32] Hu et al. had performed a prospective study on 20 patients who had two-incision THA on one hip and modified Watson-Jones THA on the other. [33] It was noted that in the early postoperative period, more patients would prefer the two-incision side to the modified Watson-Jones side. Taking the similarity of the two muscle-sparing techniques in regards to the anterior approach to the hip joint, it was postulated that the manipulation of the leg into hyperextension, external rotation, and adduction in the modified Watson-Jones technique could be the potential reason for the differences in patient's preference. We had used the modified Watson-Jones MIS-THA in more than 400 cases and had perceived similar clinical outcomes as compared with other MIS techniques. However it is usually recommended that special surgical tools, operation table, and a coordinated surgical team are the keys to success. [5,32,33]

2.13 Navigation & MIS-THA

By decreasing the surgical wound, it is difficult to visualize the surgical field in the MIS-THA. This surgical exposure is even more limited for the muscle-sparing MIS techniques. Without the help of the visualization of the surgical landmarks during operation, the operation becomes a blind method and is highly dependent on the surgeon's experiences and skillfulness. To safeguard the surgical results and to overcome the difficulty, fluoroscopy is used during the operation to provide real-time image for the verification of the implant positioning. [7,8,13,14] Fluoroscopy can also be combined with the navigation system to verify the size and position of the implants intraoperatively. By implementing the computer tomography-based or imageless navigation system with the MIS techniques, the positioning of the acetabular component could be improved by reducing the outliers with more consistent results. [3,34-36] We had adopted an imageless navigation system to the modified two-incision MIS-THA and compared the results with the use of intraoperative fluoroscopy. It was found the imageless navigation system could be a reliable tool for the cup placement as compared to intraoperative fluoroscopy. [9] However the navigation technology for the femoral component implantation is still unsatisfactory. So the navigation system cannot substitute the fluoroscopy for the original combined incision muscle-sparing MIS-THA. As described above, we had modified the two-incision technique by changing the incision direction and the patient positioning. [1,9,10] Similar to the technique described by Irving, the modified technique of two-incision THA can be safely done without the use of fluoroscopy or navigation system. [11] It is noteworthy to emphasize that the use of intraoperative fluoroscopy is not a guarantee to the safety of operation. A hairline fracture which may occur during press-fit of the implant cannot be detected by a fluoroscopy. [19] Such fracture can only be recognized by direct visualization. To overcome this difficulty, a fully porous coated stem is recommended for the muscle-sparing MIS techniques. [7,8,13,14]

2.14 Safety and complications of MIS-THA

It is assumed that the complication rates of the MIS-THA would not be lower than the conventional THA and it could be even higher if they were done by inexperienced hands especially by using the muscle-sparing techniques. The enthusiasm for the MIS-THA has declined recently because some complications have alarmed surgeons to practice more cautiously with the new MIS techniques. [13,27,29,30] The MIS-THAs, especially the multi-incision muscle-sparing techniques, are considered as unsafe with no proven benefits in clinical recovery or muscle damages. [27,28] The complications associated with the two-incision technique included higher incidence of proximal femoral fractures (2.8%) and partial, temporary injures to the lateral femoral cutaneous nerve in the so called "learning curve". [13]

However these reported complications are still not enough to conclude the MIS-THAs, muscle-sparing techniques in particular, are unsafe and associated with more complications. In the literature, the complication rates in conventional posterior or posterior mini-THA were not different with equal rates of infection, dislocation, or peroneal nerve palsy. [3,25,37,38] Ogonda et al. performed a prospectively randomized study on 219 hips by assigning them to conventional posterior or mini-posterior group. [23] The conventional group had 2 mortalities and 1 deep venous thrombosis while the mini-posterior group had 1 infection and 1 dislocation. No mortality were found in the mini-posterior group. In another study comparing conventional and mini-posterior groups, there were even higher complication rates in the conventional group. [39] By reviewing a limited number of patients retrospectively, there were higher rates of complications in the two-incision group as compared with the posterior approach group. [27,31] The two-incision group had higher complication rates (14% versus 5%) that included 4 calcar fractures, 1 dislocation, and 2 femoral nerve palsy in the 80 two-incision cases and 4 calcar fractures and 2 dislocations in the 120 posterior cases. [27] In a study of 134 hips in 125 patients by using a modified two-incision technique, there was neither major complications nor perioperative mortality. [40] Linear fractures of the femoral calcar occurred in 6 hips. Transient paresthesia of the lateral femoral cutaneous nerve was seen in 2 patients.

According to the clinical reports in the literature, the MIS-THA is associated with difficulties in the surgical techniques and should be apprehended by the surgeons to prevent complications.

2.15 Coordinating the MIS-THA team

The reasons to use the MIS techniques are to avoid unnecessary tissue destruction, to decrease tissue trauma, to increase patient's satisfaction, and to improve the clinical outcomes. However it is not enough to fulfill the goals for the early recovery by the improvement in the surgical technique alone. The surgical team, the nursing team, the physical therapy team, and the anesthesia team need to be coordinated. The multidisciplinary implementation of clinical pathway, more efficient physical therapy protocols, better anesthesia, effective postoperative pain management, and education programs are equally important as the improvement in the surgical techniques. In the author's institute, the average hospital stay after a THA is about 4 days. When the length of stay shortens, all treatments need to be accelerated without compromising the contents and qualities of medical care. In an interesting study, patients' satisfactions for a MIS-THA were highly related to the psychologic reasons. [26] Those patients who share the decision-making processes before choosing the MIS-THA will more likely take responsibility for their outcomes and cope with the treatment team.

For the improvement in the surgical techniques, it is recommended that the surgeon, the assistants, and the nursing staffs should take a training course before start. Because the adoption of a new technology needs a process of learning curve, it is also recommended that the inexperienced surgeons should work with a supervisor for about 20 cases to familiar with all the procedures. The assistants should know their roles and the steps of surgery to streamline the surgical procedures. For the MIS approach, the visualization of the surgical field is difficult for the operating surgeon. It is sometimes impossible for the assistants to see the surgical field. If the assistants can not apprehend their roles and try enthusiastically to see every anatomic detail, the difficulty for the surgeon is increased. The surgical team should use the concept of "mobile window" by moving the retractors back and forth to check the surgical anatomy one at a time. As the treatment team becomes more organized, it is more efficient to provide better quality of care and meet the interest of better patients' satisfaction.

3. Conclusion

Although the risks and benefits of MIS-THA are still inconclusive in the literature, nowadays almost all surgeons claim that they adopt some forms of MIS approach into their practice and patient care. [41-47] The reasons include the pressure from the peer groups, the patients' needs, the research and academic interests, the industrial promotion, and the surgeons' self-expectation. Information for the MIS-THA on the internet and other sources impose the MIS-THA as a metaphor of high-tech, quick-recovery, full-function, and better-satisfaction. As the conventional THA has been developed for more than 50 years and has been one of the most reliable and safe procedure in medicine, we should cautiously adopt the MIS techniques into our practice without any compromising to the gold standards of a successful THA. The fixation, the implant position, the alignment, the choice of the bearing surface, and the recreation of the normal biomechanics are the fundamental parts for long term success. The abridged incision techniques can have smaller wounds but the surgeon should not limit the incision length because most the studies indicated there were no difference in the surgical results and the clinical outcomes. For the muscle-sparing techniques, the complications are sometimes catastrophic and unacceptable in inexperienced hands in the learning curve period. The surgeons should take a cautious start by joining expert teams or taking training courses. In conclusion, the concept of MIS-THA has changed the perspectives of patient care in the hip surgery. Increasing awareness of the patients has changed the pattern of orthopedic practice. Orthopedic surgeons should take the full responsibility and master their most familiar and comfortable technique of THA. They should also adopt the MIS-THA into their practice, in the best interests of the patients, to provide long-lasting clinical outcomes and minimize trauma to the patients.

4. References

[1] Chen DW, Hu CC, Chang YH, Yang WE, Lee MS. Comparison of clinical outcome in primary total hip arthroplasty by conventional anterolateral transgluteal or 2-incision approach. J Arthroplast 2009;24:528-532.

[2] Sculco TP, Jordan LC. The mini-incision approach to total hip arthroplasty. Instr Course Lect 2004;53:141-147.

[3] Dorr LD, Maheshwari AV, Long WT, Wan Z, Sirianni LE. Early pain relief and function after posterior minimally invasive and conventional total hip arthroplasty. A prospective, randomized, blinded study. J Bone Joint Surg Am 2007;89:1153-1160.

[4] Swanson TV. Early results of 1000 consecutive, posterior, single-incision minimally invasive surgery total hip arthroplasties. J Arthroplast 2005;20:Suppl 26-32.

[5] Bertin KC, Röttinger H. Anterolateral mini-incision hip replacement surgery. A modified Watson-Jones approach. Clin Orthop 2004;429:248-255.

[6] Lovell TP. Single-incision direct anterior approach for total hip arthroplasty using a standard operating table. J Arthroplast 2008;23:S64-S68.

[7] Berger RA. Total hip arthroplasty using the minimally invasive two-incision approach. Clin Orthop 2003;417:232-241.

[8] Berger RA, Jacobs JJ, Meneghini RM, Valle CD, Paprosky W, Rosenberg AG. Rapid rehabilitation and recovery with minimally invasive total hip arthroplasty. Clin Orthop 2004;429:239-247.

[9] Lee MS, Kuo CH, Senan V, Chen WJ, Chen LH, Ueng SWN. Two-incision total hip replacement: Intraoperative fluoroscopy versus imageless navigation. Hip International 2006;16 (Suppl): S35-S41.

[10] Chou SW, Ueng SWN, Lee MS. Muscular recovery of hip flexors and extensors after two-incision total hip arthroplasty. Chang Gung Med J 2008;31(6):576-582.

[11] Irving JF. Direct two-incision total hip replacement without fluoroscopy. Orthop Clin N Am 2004;35:173-181.

[12] Kennon RE, Keggi JM, Wetmore RS, Zatorski LE, Huo MH. Keggi KJ. Total hip arthroplasty through a minimally invasive anterior surgical approach. J Bone Joint Surg Am 2003;85(Suppl 4): 39-48.

[13] Archibeck MJ, White RE Jr. Learning curve for the two-incision total hip replacement. Clin Orthop 2004;429:232-238.

[14] Berry DJ, Berger RA, Callaghan JJ, Dorr LD, Duwelius PJ, Hartzband MA, Lieberman JR, Mears DC. American orthopaedic association symposium: minimally invasive total hip arthroplasty: development, early results, and a critical analysis. J Bone Joint Surg Am 2003;85: 2235-2246.

[15] Solberg BD, Moon CN, Franco DP. Use of a trochanteric flip osteotomy improves outcomes in Pipkin IV fractures. Clin Orthop 2009;467:929-933.

[16] Mardones R, Gonazalez C, Cabanela ME, Trousdale RT, Berry DJ. Extended femoral osteotomy for revision of hip arthroplasty. Results and complications. J Arthroplast 2005;20:79-83.

[17] Hardinge K. The direct lateral approach to the hip. J Bone Joint Surg Br. 1982;64:17-19.

[18] Picado CH, Garcia FL, Marques W, Jr. Damage to the superior gluteal nerve after direct lateral approach to the hip. Clin Orthop 2007;455:209-211.

[19] Hu CC, Yang WE, Chang YH, Chen DWC, Ueng SWN, Lee MS. Fluoroscopy can not recognize intraoperative fracture in patients receiving two-incision total hip arthroplasty. J Arthoplast 2008;23:1031-1036.

[20] Learmonth ID, Allen PE. The omega lateral approach to the hip. J Bone Joint Surg 1996;78-B:559-561.

[21] Bohler N, Hipmair G. The minimal invasive surgery anterior approach with supine patient positioning: a step-wise introduction of technique. Hip International 2006;16(Suppl4):48-53.

[22] Matta J, Shahrdar C, Ferfuson T. Single-incision anterior approach for total hip arthroplasty on an orthoaedic table. Clin Orthop 2005;441:115-124.

[23] Ogonda L, Wilson R, Archbold P, Lawlor M, Humphreys P, O'Brien S, Beverland D. A minimal-incision technique in total hip arthroplasty does not improve early postoperative outcomes. A prospective, randomized, controlled trial. J Bone Joint Surg Am 2005;87(4):701-710.

[24] Bennett D, Ogonda L, Elliott D, Humphreys L, Lawlor M, Beverland D. Comparison of immediate postoperative walking ability in patients receiving minimally invasive and standard-incision hip arthroplasty. A prospective blinded study. J Arthoplasty 2007;22:490-495.

[25] Kim YH. Comparison of primary total hip arthroplasties performed with a minimally invasive technique or a standard technique. A prospective and randomized study. J Arthroplasty 2006;21:1092-1098.

[26] Dorr LD, Thomas D, Long WT, Polatin PB, Sirianni LE. Psychologic reasons for patients preferring minimally invasive total hip arthroplasty. Clin Orthop 2007;458:94-100.

[27] Pagnano MW, Leone J, Lewallen DG, Hanssen AD. Two-incision THA had modest outcomes and some substantial complications. Clin Orthop 2005;441:86-90.

[28] Mardones R, Pagnano MW, Nemanich JP, Trousdale RT. Muscle damage after total hip arthroplasty done with the two-incision and mini-posterior techniques. Clin Orthop 2005;441;63-67.

[29] Fehring TK, Mason JB. Catastrophic complications of minimally invasive hip surgery. A series of three cases. J Bone Joint Surg Am 2005;87:711-714.

[30] Feinblatt JS, Berend KR, Lombardi AV Jr. Severe symptomatic heterotopic ossification and dislocation: a complication after two-incision minimally invasive total hip arthroplasty. J Arthroplasty 2005;20(6):802-806.

[31] Duwelius PJ, Burkhart RL, Hayhurst JO, Moller H, Butler JBV. Comparison of the 2-incision and mini-incision posterior total hip arthroplasty technique. A retrospective match-pair control technique. J Arthroplast 2007;22:48-56.

[32] Laffosse JM, Accadbled F, Molinier F, Chiron P, Hocine B, Puget J. Anterolateral mini-invasive versus posterior mini-invasive approach for primary total hip replacement. Comparison of exposure and implant positioning. Arch Orthop Trauma Surg 2008;128(4):363-369.

[33] Hu CC, Chern JS, Hsieh PH, Shih CH, Ueng SWN, Lee MS. Two-incision versus modified Watson-Jones total hip arthroplasty in the same patient – a prospective study on clinical outcomes and patient's preference. Chang Gung Med J 2011 (In Press).

[34] Wixson RL, MacDonald MA. Total hip arthroplasty through a minimal posterior approach using imageless computer-assisted hip navigation. J Arthroplasty 2005;20,Suppl 3:51-56.

[35] Parratte S, Argenson JA. Validation and usefulness of a computer-assisted cup-positioning system in total hip arthroplasty. A prospective, randomized, control study. J Bone Joint Surg Am 2007;89:494-499.

[36] Haaker RGA, Tiedjen K, Ottersbach A, Rubenthaler F, Stockheim M, Stiehl JB. Comparison of conventional versus computer-navigated acetabular component insertion. J Arthroplast 2007;22:151-159.

[37] Geubbels ELPE, Wille JC, Nagelkerke NJD, Vandenbroucke-Grauls CMJE, Grobbee DE, de Boer AS. Hospital-related determinants for surgical-site infection following hip arthroplasty. Infect Control Hosp Epidemiol 2005;26:435-441.

[38] Ridgeway S, Wilson J, Charlet A, Kafatos G, Pearson A, Coello R. Infection of the surgical site after arthroplasty of the hip. J Bone Joint Surg Br 2005;87 (6):844-50.

[39] Khan RJK, Fick D, Khoo P, Yao F, Nivbrant B, Wood D. Less invasive total hip arthroplasty: description of a new technique. J Arthroplast 2006; 21:1038-1046.

[40] Lu ML, Chou SW, Yang WE, Senan V, Hsieh PH, Shih HN, Lee MS. Hospital course and early clinical outcomes of two-incision total hip arthroplasty. Chang Gung Med J 2007;30(6):513-520.

[41] Wright JM, Crockett HC, Delgado S, Lyman S, Madsen M, Sculco TP. Mini-incision for total hip arthroplasty. A prospective, controlled investigation with 5-year follow-up evaluation. J Arthroplasty 2004;19(5):538-545.

[42] Siguier T, Siguier M, Brumpt B. Mini-incision anterior approach does not increase dislocation rate. A study of 1037 total hip replacements. Clin Orthop 2004;426:164-173.

[43] de Beer J, Petruccelli D, Zalzal P, Winemaker MJ. Single incision minimally invasive total hip arthroplasty: length doesn't matter. J Arthroplasty 2004;19(8):945-950.

[44] Howell JR, Masri BA, Duncan CP. Minimally invasive versus standard incision anterolateral hip replacement: a comparative study. Orthop Clin North Am 2004;35(2):153-162.

[45] Asayama I, Kinsey TL, Mahoney OM. Two-year experience using a limited-incision direct lateral approach in total hip arthroplasty. J Arthroplast 2006;21:1083-1091.

[46] Meneghini RM, Smits SA. Early discharge and recovery with three minimally invasive total hip arthroplasty approaches. Clin Orthop 2009;467:1431-1437.

[47] Labovitch RS, Bozic KJ, Hansen E. An evaluation of information available on the internet regarding minimally invasive hip arthroplasty. J Arthroplast 2006;21:1-5.

6

The Effect of Drainage After Hip Arthroplasty

Andrej Strahovnik and Samo K. Fokter

General and Teaching Hospital Celje
Slovenia

1. Introduction

Closed suction drainage is a routinely used method in all fields of surgery. The idea to drain a wound is quite old. Supposedly, Hippocrates had already used a wooden tube to drain the operative wound (Levy, 1984). In orthopaedic surgery, Waugh and Stinchfield were the first who popularized the method of draining. Their preference to draining was based on their retrospective study, where they observed the incidence of wound infection after various orthopaedic procedures (Waugh & Stinchfield, 1961). The group of 100 patients with closed suction drainage was compared with a similar group (identical procedure, same comorbidities and the same surgeon) of 100 patients without the drainage. Wound infection occurred in 1% of patients with closed suction drainage and in 3% of patients without the drainage. They also noted that the post-operative rehabilitation was quicker if they drained the operated joint after an arthroplasty. Even though the difference in incidence of wound infection was not statistically significant, they concluded that a more benign postoperative course can be expected if the drains are used.

After that, the use of drains quickly spread in all areas of orthopaedic surgery. It seemed logical to drain the operative wound. Exposed intramedullary canal and trabecular bone make it difficult to create a perfect hemostasis. A hematoma inevitably forms which increases the pressure on the surrounding tissues. Increased pressure impairs blood flow and healing of the operative wound. Additionally, a hematoma is also a good culture medium for bacteria (Cheung et al., 2008; Parvizi et al., 2007). The function of phagocytic cells to eliminate these bacteria in hematoma is weakened. The first reason for this weakened elimination is that phagocytic cells have a hardened access to the bacteria in the hematoma. Secondly, due to the low level of opsonic proteins in hematoma, the destruction capacity of phagocytic cells is damaged (Alexander et al., 1976). Therefore, in order to prevent the infection of the surgical wound, it appears logical to drain the wound to avoid or at least reduce the formation of hematoma.

New studies have emerged at the end of the 20th century. These studies have questioned the logical mechanism of drainage and the use of drainage in hip arthroplasty. There are several potential adverse effects from draining. Drain tubes may become contaminated and allow a retrograde migration of the skin bacteria around the wound. In addition, drains may be inadvertently sutured to surrounding tissues and are difficult to remove post-operatively. Furthermore, drains may increase the amount of blood loss and increase the need for transfusion. The findings from these new studies have convinced many surgeons to change their routine and re-think the need for drainage in total hip arthroplasty.

2. Literature search methods

All randomized controlled trials that compared closed suction drainage to no-drainage after elective hip arthroplasty were searched. Additionally, studies that could provide further information on relevant aspects of drainage (eg. relative amount of drainage in the first 24 hours, hematoma size estimation using one or two drain tubes, bacterial growth on suction drain tips, etc.) were included. Trials involving other than elective hip arthroplasty (arthroplasty for fracture treatment) were excluded. The following search terms were used in Pubmed database: "drainage hip arthroplasty", "drains hip arthroplasty", "serous drainage hip arthroplasty". Two authors independently examined all articles that were obtained with this search strategy. Articles were assessed for relevance and handpicked. Differences between authors were resolved by discussion.

The selection procedure resulted in 6 studies directly comparing the use of closed suction drainage to un-drained wound closure (Murphy & Scott, 1993; Kim et al., 1998; Widman et al., 2002; Della Valle et al., 2004; Johansson et al., 2005; Walmsley et al., 2005). The basic information about the studies is depicted in Table 1.

Study	Drained group (hips, n)	Un-drained group (hips, n)	Number of drains (n)	Time of drain removal (h)	Follow-up
Murphy & Scott, 1993	20	20	2	24	10 days
Kim et al., 1998	48	48	2	24	1 year
Widman et al., 2002	10	12	2	24	NA*
Della Valle et al., 2004	53	51	2	next morning	3 months
Johansson et al., 2005	54	51	NA	NA	2 months
Walmsley et al., 2005	282	295	1	24	3 years

* data not available

Table 1. Studies with a direct comparison of drained group to un-drained group.

Seven studies, which in addition to groups with and without closed suction drainage after hip arthroplasty, compared groups with different interventions (eg. additional group after knee arthroplasty; two drained groups, one with 24-hour drainage, the other with 48-hour drainage; two drained groups, one with autologous blood transfusion drain, one with conventional closed suction drainage) were also included in a review (Beer et al., 1991; Ritter et al., 1994; Ovadia et al., 1997; Niskanen et al., 2000; Kumar et al., 2007; Strahovnik et al., 2010; Cheung et al., 2010). Characteristics of those studies are presented in Table 2.

Three more studies were included with relevant data on infection of the surgical wound, one study with data on hematoma size and two studies on the prolonged serous secretion from the surgical wound (Willett et al., 1988; Sørensen & Sørensen, 1991; Overgaard et al., 1993; Parrini et al., 1988; Wood et al., 2007; Patel et al., 2007).

Study	Drained group (hips, n)	Un-drained group (hips, n)	Additional intervention - arm
Beer at al., 1991	12	12	two knee groups
Ritter at al., 1994	78	62	two knee groups
Ovadia et al., 1997	18	12	two knee groups
Niskanen et al., 2000	27	31	two knee groups
Kumar et al., 2007	19	15	two knee groups
Strahovnik et al., 2010	46	42	group with 48h drainage
Cheung et al., 2010	52	48	group with autologous transfusion drain

Table 2. Studies with additional research arm(s).

Different aspects of wound healing with or without drainage after hip arthroplasty were reviewed and compared among the selected studies. The effectivenes of drainage with regard to those aspects is discussed under the following heading. Drainage also has an unwanted side effect that was not present in the un-drained groups, which is reported in a later heading as a complication.

3. Effectiveness of drainage in total hip arthroplasty

The impact of drainage on the bacterial growth and wound infection was regarded as the most important outcome. The drainage influence on the size of hematoma, the healing of the surgical wound, the need for transfusion and hospital stay were also reported in most of the studies.

3.1 Bacterial growth and wound infection

No significant difference in the occurrence of wound infection was found in the studies that were directly comparing patients whose wounds were drained and patients with un-drained wounds. If infection was present, it was regarded as superficial in the majority of cases. Deep wound infection was very rare or none. Results are summarized in Table 3.

Other studies that were comparing groups with additional intervention, as well as drainage and no-drainage groups after hip arthroplasty, also could not show any differences in wound infection.

Altogether, there were 30 out of 719 patients with wound infection (superficial and deep) in the drained groups, and 27 out of 699 patients in the no-drained groups (relative risk 1.08; 95% confidence interval 0.65 – 1.80).

Wound infection is a serious complication after elective hip arthroplasty. It should be regarded as the most important reported outcome. The problem is that the occurrence of wound infection, either superficial or deep, is very low. In order to achieve the required power and still get a clinically significant difference between groups, a large number of patients would need to be included in a study. In a hypothetical scenario, where we would have, for example, a 6% incidence of wound infection in the drained group, and a 3% incidence in the no-drained group (no published study reported such a big difference), and the power of a study 0.8, we would need at least 312 patients to achieve a significant difference with probability less than 0.05.

The only single study that included a sufficient number of patients was from Walmsley et al. They found the rate of superficial infection 2.9% in the drained group and 4.8% in the un-drained group. The rate of deep wound infection was 0.4% in the drained group and 0.7% in the un-drained group. The differences in the incidence of wound infection were not statistically significant. The only existent meta-analysis on hip arthroplasty managed to pool 711 patients with drained wounds and 704 patients with un-drained wounds (Parker et al., 2008). The pooled results indicated that there was no significant difference between the wounds treated with a drain and those treated without a drain with respect to the occurrence of wound infection.

Study	Wound infection - deep&superficial (n/N)		Deep wound infection (n)	
	Drained group	Un-drained group	Drained group	Un-drained group
Beer et al., 1991	0/12	0/12	0	0
Murphy & Scott, 1993	1/20	0/20	NA	NA
Ritter et al., 1994	0/78	0/62	0	0
Ovadia et al., 1997	0/18	0/12	0	0
Kim et al., 1998	0/48	0/48	NA	NA
Niskanen et al., 2000	1/27	1/31	0	0
Widman et al., 2002	1/10	1/12	1	1
Della Valle et al., 2004	2/53	0/51	0	0
Johansson et al., 2005	3/54	2/51	0	0
Walmsley et al., 2005	19/282	23/295	1	2
Kumar et al., 2007	0/19	0/15	0	0
Strahovnik et al., 2010	1/46	0/42	0	0
Cheung et al., 2010	2/52	0/48	0	0

Table 3. Incidence of wound infection.

Another problem with reporting incidence of wound infection is limited follow-up. Many studies followed patients only until first clinical control. This may have resulted in an underreporting of not only the infection rate but of several other outcomes as well (eg. re-operation rate).

We can conclude that drainage does not have a clinically relevant effect on wound infection after hip arthroplasty.

3.1.1 Connection between wound infection and duration of drainage

The supposedly beneficial effect of drainage on the bacterial growth in the drained hematoma was actually one of the first assumptions to become questioned. Willett et al. performed a study with 120 patients after hip arthroplasty (Willett et al., 1988). They implied a connection between wound infection and the duration of drainage. Even though the correlation did not reach the statistical significance, the authors recommended removal of drains 24 hours after the operation. Drainage after 24 hours did not reduce the size of hematoma, but it did increase the chance of bacterial infection.

Similarly, Sørensen and Sørensen also investigated the relation between bacterial growth and duration of drainage (Sørensen & Sørensen, 1991). They prospectively followed 489 patients after various orthopaedic operations. They showed that signs of wound infection and drain tip cultures were significantly more often positive, if the drainage lasted more than 6 days. The explanation they offered was that the drain allows the bacteria on the skin around the wound to retrogradely migrate.

On the other hand, another study between drain tip cultures and the duration of drainage did not show any statistically significant correlation (Overgaard et al., 1993). The authors commented that this unexpected lack of correlation might be explained with a relatively short duration of drainage in their study (maximum 3 days). They also noticed that most of the drainage occurred within first 12 hours, and hence also recommended to remove the drains rather sooner than later.

Additional studies on relationship between the duration of drainage and bacterial infection were performed (Drinkwater & Neil, 1995; Erceg & Becić K, 2008; Rowe et al., 1993). A general consensus was gradually formed that the optimal time to remove the drains in hip arthroplasty would be 24 hours after the operation. Drainage after first 24 hours does not evacuate significant amount of blood and only increases the chance of bacterial retrograde migration.

3.2 Hematoma size

Several studies evaluated the size of hematoma after hip arthroplasty (Murphy & Scott, 1993; Kim et al., 1998; Widman et al., 2002). Hematoma size can be evaluated using different methods, but none of them is very accurate. Most of the studies used a formula which uses pre-operative and post-operative hematocrit values to calculate hidden blood loss (hematoma). In some studies an ultrasound examination of the thigh was used, in order to measure the thickness of blood mantle around the prosthesis. Other methods have also been used, such as a scintigraphy with labeled erythrocytes or a simple tape measurement of the thigh circumference.

In one study a calculated hidden loss in the wound was compared between a group with drainage and a group without the drainage (Murphy & Scott, 1993). Hematoma in the drained group was not smaller. The authors explained this unexpected result with a tamponade effect mechanism. The tamponade effect refers to the fact that the bleeding in the wound continues until the pressure in the wound increases. In order to achieve the critical pressure, enough bleeding must occur to fill out the space (dead space) around the prosthesis. Since the tissues around the hip prosthesis are relatively rigid and immobile, the suction from the drain does not reduce the space around prosthesis (dead space). In other words, regardless the wound is drained or not, enough bleeding into the wound must occur to create the tamponade effect. Furthermore, a drain enlarges the dead space for the amount of space of a drain tube and a drain device. Therefore, even more blood must be lost to achieve the tamponade effect, if a drain is used. Paradoxically, drains therefore increase the blood loss after the operation.

Widman et al. used a more objective method of determining the hematoma size (Widman et al., 2002). They used a scintigraphy with labeled erythrocytes to compare a group of patients with two-drain drainage to a group of patients without the drainage. The hematoma size was quantitatively measured using SPECT (single photon emission computed tomography). Even though a smaller hematoma was found when two drains were used, the difference between patients with drained wounds and patients with un-drained wounds was not statistically significant. Patients with drainage also lost more blood and more often required blood transfusion in the postoperative period. The authors´ interpretation was consistent with a tamponade effect theory.

On the other hand, Kim et al. routinely used ultrasound to assess the size of wound hematoma on the sixth or seventh day after the surgery (Kim et al., 1998). The wound hematoma was classified as none, small or large, according to the thickness of the hypoechogenic density along the region of the wound. Thirteen drained wounds (27.1%) and 26 non-drained wounds (54.2%) had large hematomas; large hematomas were significantly more often present in patients without the drainage. In addition, 13 wounds with closed suction drainage (27.1%) and 4 wounds without the drainage (8.3%) did not have hematomas, which was also statistically significant difference. The possible explanation the authors offered was that the use of suction drains may not evacuate hematomas completely in the hip joint, and that small hematomas re-accumulate in the hip joint after the drain is removed.

Another study examined the hematoma size using an ultra-sonographic evaluation (Parrini et al., 1988). Within 82 patients after total hip arthroplasty, a comparison between patients with two drains and patients with one drain was made. A hematoma in the wound was always present, regardless to the number of drains. However, the authors did found the hematoma to be significantly smaller in patients, where two drains were used instead of one.

We also performed a study where we compared 3 groups: a group without drainage, a group with 24-hour drainage and a group with 48-hour drainage. A semi-quantitative estimation of the wound hematoma size was performed with measurements of the operated thigh circumference. Measurements of the thigh circumference were routinely performed before and after elective total hip arthroplasty. In the un-drained group, the change of thigh circumference significantly increased in the post-operative period, when compared with the change in both drained groups. Most of the increase of thigh circumference occurred within first 48 hours after the procedure. Our results were consistent with findings of both previous studies. The use of drainage slightly decreases hematoma size in the post-operative period. However, the drains do not evacuate hematomas completely, and hematomas re-accumulate to a certain extent after the drains are removed.

3.3 Healing of the surgical wound

There are few studies thoroughly describing wound healing parameters, such as bruising of the wound area and persistent drainage from the wound. No study reported any serious healing complications (eg. necrosis of the skin around the wound). Most of the studies described healing as uneventful in either drained or un-drained groups and did not notice any difference.

3.3.1 Bruising of the wound area

There is only one study reporting bruising around the wound area after hip arthroplasty. Kim et.al measured the area of bluish discoloration around the wound site. The ecchymosis was present in 11 hips from the un-drained group, as opposed to 3 hips from the drained group (p<0.05). They recommended the routine use of suction drains after primary total hip arthroplasty to reduce ecchymosis around the wound. Other studies did not specifically report the bruising around the wound area.

3.3.2 Persistent drainage from the wound site

There are two types of prolonged drainage in hip arthroplasty. The first type occurs in the surgical wound and can happen whether the wound is drained or not. The second type of drainage occurs only in drained wounds, at the drain site after the drain is removed.

The drainage from the surgical wound usually starts on the first post-operative day and rarely lasts for more than a couple of days. The drainage is usually bloody. This type of drainage is more frequent if the wound is not drained. Kim et al. found persistent drainage from the surgical wound in 3 of 48 wounds with suction drains and 11 of 48 wounds without suction drains. Other studies do not specifically report the drainage from the wound site.

Sometimes a later secretion from the surgical wound develops which is serous in nature and may last longer. This type of serous secretion has been linked to the development of superficial surgical site infection and deep wound infection (Saleh et al., 2002). Serous secretion allows an open communication between the deep layers of the surgical wound and the skin. The longer this communication exists, the more chance there is for migration of bacteria from the skin.

Two studies have analyzed risk factors that predispose to the longer duration of prolonged serous secretion from the wound site. Wood et al. associated time to dryness of the surgical wound with: wound length, body mass index (BMI) and estimated volume of blood in the dissected tissues (Wood et al., 2007). Patel et al. found that prolonged wound drainage correlated with: morbid obesity (BMI $\geq 40 kg/m^2$), increased volume of drain output and use of low-molecular-weight heparin (Patel et al., 2007). In both studies, the length of hospital stay was significantly increased in patients with prolonged drainage. Patel et al. also stated that each day of prolonged wound drainage increased the risk of wound infection by 42% following a total hip arthroplasty.

3.3.3 Re-operation for wound healing complication

There was no statistically significant difference in the re-operation rate between the groups (Table 4).

Study	Drained group (n/N)	Un-drained group (n/N)
Kim et al., 1998	0/48	0/48
Della Valle et al., 2004	1/53	0/51
Johansson et al., 2005	0/54	0/51
Walmsley et al., 2005	1/282	0/295
Strahovnik et al., 2010	1/46	0/42
Cheung et al., 2010	0/52	0/48

Table 4. Re-operation due to wound healing complications.

3.4 Post-operative range of hip motion

There was only one study numerically reporting post-operative range of motion. Kim et al. reported no extension lag in either group at the 2-month follow-up. Mean flexion reached 90° in the drained group and 95° in the group without drainage.

3.4.1 Need for re-enforcement of the dressing

Since more patients without closed suction drainage have a persistent drainage from the surgical wound, more wounds need to be re-enforced in the early post-operative period.

Several studies have reported a greater need for re-enforcement of the dressing in the un-drained groups (Table 5). Two of them have found a statistically significant difference between drained and un-drained groups (Kim et al. 1998; Strahovnik et al., 2010).

Study	Drained group (n/N)	Un-drained group (n/N)
Kim et al., 1998	3/48	11/48
Niskanen et al., 2000	1/27	4/31
Della Valle et al., 2004	6/53	10/ 51
Strahovnik et al., 2010	2/46	20/42

Table 5. Studies with reported need for re-enforcement of the dressing.

3.5 Need for blood transfusion

The majority of included studies evaluated the need for transfusion. The need for transfusion is an easily measured parameter and could be one of the most important evidences of the tamponade effect theory. One point needs to be addressed with regard to the transfusion needs as an outcome measure. Different transfusion triggers were used in analyzed studies. Some authors used an absolute hemoglobin cutoff point, with values bellow that point necessitating a blood transfusion. Others used various recommended algorithms or they simply treated each patient and their requirements for allogeneic blood on an individual basis. In some studies the transfusion algorithm was not well described. This heterogeneity of transfusion policies could not be eliminated in the analysis. Different transfusion triggers among and even within the studies reduce the reliability of the need for transfusion as an outcome measure.

There is a trend in the need for more blood transfusion if drains are used in total hip arthroplasty. Many studies showed the increased need for transfusion in patients with drained wounds but only studies by Walmsley et al., Strahovnik et al. and Cheung et al. showed that the need for transfusion was significantly more often required in patients with drainage (Table 6).

Study	Patients transfused		p
	Drained group (n/N)	Un-drained group (n/N)	
Ovadia et al., 1997	9/18	2/12	0.06
Widman et al., 2002	9/10	6/12	0.07
Della Valle et al. 2004	21/53	18/51	0.7
Johansson et al. 2005	36/54	28/51	0.3
Walmsley et al., 2005	93/282	78/295	0.042
Kumar et al., 2007	13/19	10/15	0.13
Strahovnik et al., 2010	22/46	30/42	0.024
Cheung et al., 2010	19/52	6/48	0.02

Table 6. Incidence of transfusion needed in drained and un-drained groups.

For included studies in Table 6, the relative risk for transfusion in patients with closed suction drainage opposed to patients without drainage was 1.23 (95% confidence interval 1.05 – 1.44). Accordingly, more units of red cell concentrates were given to patients in the drained groups (Table 7). However, when there was a need for blood transfusion, patients received approximately the same amount of red cell concentrates, regardless of the fact whether the wound was drained or not.

Study	Units of blood given (n)/number of patients)	
	Drained group	Un-drained group
Ovadia et al., 1997	13U/9	3U/2
Johanson et al., 2005	110U/36	69U/28
Cheung et al., 2010	36U/19	11U/6

Table 7. Number of units of red cell concentrates given.

Results are consistent with the tamponade effect theory. Drains evacuate the blood that would otherwise be required to achieve the sufficient intra-wound pressure in order to stop the bleeding. The more blood is evacuated, the greater the need for transfusion.

3.6 Hospital stay
With the exception of studies by Cheung et al. and Della Valle et al., which reported a significant difference between the drained and un-drained group, other studies did not found any differences in hospital stay after hip arthroplasty. Drainage does not seem to directly affect the duration of hospitalization. Mean values of hospital stay ranged from 5 to 10 days in both of groups (Table 8). Within the two studies with statistically significant difference in hospital stay, only the difference of one day could be regarded as clinically relevant. Authors interpreted that this difference in length of stay is most likely a reflection of the greater amount of time it took for the drained wounds to become dry. However, wound-healing disturbances in the drained group might have been related to an allogeneic transfusion (in this particular study, the transfusion rates were much higher in patients with closed suction drainage), and not to drain usage per se.

Study	Drained group (days)	Un-drained group (days)	p
Ovadia et al., 1997	10	8.3	0.06
Della Valle et al., 2004	5.1	4.7	0.01
Walmsley et al., 2005	10	10	NA
Kumar et al., 2007	8.9	8.4	0.32
Strahovnik et al., 2010	7	7	0.55
Cheung et al., 2010	7	6	0.03

Table 8. Average hospitalization time.

Namely, there seems to be a relation between allogeneic transfusion and disturbances in wound healing, which in turn affects the hospital stay. The mechanism by which wound-healing disturbances and length of hospital stay are related are still unclear (Weber et al., 2005). First possible explanation is a direct effect of tissue hypoxia as a consequence of decreased values of hemoglobin in the post-operative period. However, in a clinical study, the anemia was present in groups without closed suction drains as well and did not affect wound healing. This effect seems, therefore, unlikely. The alternative explanation might be the immuno-modulatory effect of allogeneic blood. Experimental studies have shown that the immuno-modulatory effects of allogeneic blood transfusion might lead to a decrease in proangiogenic factors that are essential for wound healing (eg. interleukin 8). Allogeneic blood tranfusion might therefore induce a small but significant delay in wound healing. Since drainage seems to affect the transfusion rates, it might also indirectly influence the hospital stay.

3.7 Cost analysis

Three studies analyzed the costs of drainage in total hip arthroplasty. The savings of the cost of closed suction units (hemovacs) was reported if drains were omitted in hip arthroplasty (Ritter et al., 1994; Kim et al., 1998). Della Valle et al. stated that the additional sum could be saved due to a shorter hospital stay in patients without closed suction drainage.

4. Complications of drainage

The unwanted side effects, which occur only in patients where closed suction drainage was used, are described here. The possible deleterious effects of drains on wound infection, need for transfusion and hospital stay were already discussed in the previous section.

4.1 Prolonged drainage from the drain site

Prolonged drainage from the wound is the second type of prolonged drainage in hip arthroplasty. This type of persistent, prolonged drainage occurs on the drain site after the drain is removed. It is more frequent (up to 50% of patients with drainage) and usually more persistent.

Our own study showed that prolonged secretion from the drain site typically started on the third post-operative day and lasted for four days on the average. Prolonged secretion rarely lasted more than 14 days. In addition, the incidence and duration of prolonged serous secretion were comparable between the group with 24-hour drainage and the group with 48-hour drainage. The greatest proportion of patients with active secretion in both groups was present on the 5th post-operative day (Figure 1).

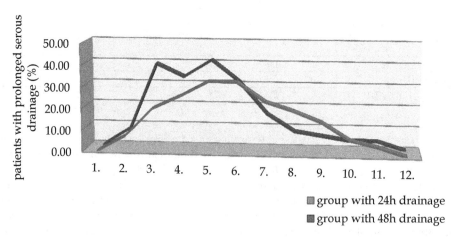

Fig. 1. Proportion of patients with active secretion from the drain site in groups with drainage.

Division of prolonged drainage on the drainage from the wound site and the drainage from the drain site is arbitrary. The cause of drainage is the same regardless on the location. The drainage is linked to a hematoma that develops around the prosthesis. At first, the drainage is bloody, but later turns to serous fluid as the red cells in hematoma sediment. Since the hematoma in the wound is always present whether the drain is present or not, prolonged drainage is always possible. In the un-drained wounds, the drainage can occur through the incision plane, especially if the fascia was not meticulously sutured. In case of a drained wound, the hematoma drains through the drain tube. After the drains are removed, the hematoma may drain through the un-healed drain canal (Figure 2). The drainage stops with the healing of the canal.

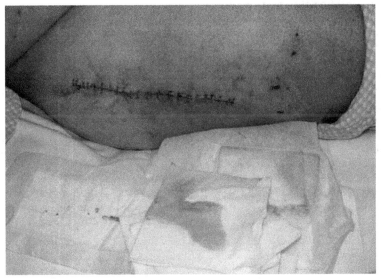

Fig. 2. Wound with prolonged serous secretion through an un-healed drain canal.

In conclusion, late secretion from the drain site is frequent and usually spontaneously resolves within 3 to 4 days. Longer secretion, especially longer than 14 days, predisposes to the development of wound infection. Careful observation, supervised regular changing of the dressings and even revision surgery may be necessary to stop the secretion in persistent cases.

5. Additional methods to influence the drainage

Several additional methods can be applied to decrease the bleeding and hence drainage from the surgical wound. The use of hypotensive anesthesia is well established in orthopaedic surgery. A thorough hemostasis at the end of the procedure is also a prerequisite in hip arthroplasty. Some advocate the use of pneumatic wound compression as a method of reducing post-operative bleeding.

Recently, pharmacological strategies have become of interest to decrease excessive blood lost. An intravenous administration of tranexamic acid before hip arthroplasty significantly decreased peri-operative bleeding (Ekbäck et al., 2000; Singh et al., 2010). Tranexamic acid seems to be a cost-effective and safe mean of minimizing blood loss and reduction in hemoglobin concentrations as well as the need for allogeneic blood transfusion, without increasing the risk of thromboembolic events.

6. Conclusion

Common practice of draining has recently become questioned in orthopaedic surgery. Many randomized trials have been performed, trying to provide a definite answer about the efficacy of draining. Even though the number of trials on the topic is considerable, very few have good methodology which would allow us to draw reliable conclusions. The majority of studies were underpowered for accurate assessment of most important outcomes (eg. wound infection, re-operation rate). Many of them also had a short follow-up period, which allows underreporting of important medical events.

Having already realized the drawbacks of studies in the literature, Parker et al. carried out a meta-analysis. However, due to enormous variety of methods in the orthopaedic community, it is very hard to find studies with homogeneous group of patients. The common denominator of selected studies in their meta-analysis as well as in this review was an elective total hip arthroplasty. Numerous other parameters that could affect the outcomes could not be controlled. For example, even though patients underwent the same procedure, the surgical approach was not uniform in the included studies. Patients varied also in several other parameters: diagnosis, number of drains placed, location of drains, duration of drainage, type of prosthesis, use of thromboprophylaxis, compression of the thigh, trigger for transfusion, post-operative rehabilitation regime, patient's discharge trigger and follow-up period. All these parameters were not uniform or were not even reported.

An evaluation of most of the reported outcomes was given in our review. Since a simple division into pro draining and con draining could not be made for the majority of the observed outcomes, we summarized our conclusions about outcomes as a degree of certainty with regard to the evidence available. Our conclusions are presented in Table 9.

outcome	in favor of		draining	in disfavor of	
	definite evidence	some evidence	undecided	some evidence	definite evidence
Wound infection			X		
Hematoma formation			X		
Bruising of the wound		X			
Drainage from wound		X			
Re-operation			X		
Rehabilitation			X		
Need for re-enforcement		X			
Need for transfusion				X	
Hospital stay				X	
Cost					X
Drainage from drain site					X

Table 9. List of outcomes and categorization in terms of pro et contra draining.

In conclusion, randomized studies have shown that closed suction drainage is not necessary in total hip arthroplasty and may be, in some aspects, even deleterious. However, due to the heterogeneity of practice, every surgeon must combine his own routine with the decision to drain.

7. References

Alexander JW, Korelitz J, Alexander NS. (1976). Prevention of wound infections. A case for closed suction drainage to remove wound fluids deficient in opsonic proteins. *Am J Surg*, Vol. 132, No. 1, (July 1976), pp. 59-63, ISSN 0002-9610

Beer KJ, Lombardi AV, Mallory TH, Vaughn BK. (1991). The efficacy of suction drains after routine total joint arthroplasty. *J Bone Joint Surg Am*, Vol. 73, No. 4, (April 1991), pp. 584-586, ISSN 0021-9355

Cheung EV, Sperling JW, Cofield RH. (2008). Infection associated with hematoma formation after shoulder arthroplasty. *Clin Orthop Relat Res*, Vol. 466, No. 6, (June 2008), pp. 1363-1367, ISSN 0009-921X

Cheung G, Carmont MR, Bing AJ,Kuiper JH, Alcock RJ, Graham NM. (2010). No drain, autologous transfusion drain or suction drain? A randomised prospective study in total hip replacement surgery of 168 patients. *Acta Orthop Belg*, Vol. 76, No. 5, (October 2010), pp. 619-627, ISSN 0001-6462

Della Valle AG, Slullitel G, Vestri R, Comba F, Buttaro M, Piccaluga F. (2004). No need for routine closed suction drainage in elective arthroplasty of the hip. A prospective randomized trial in 104 operations. *Acta Orthop Scand*, Vol. 75, No. 1, (February 2004), pp. 30-33, ISSN 0001-6470

Drinkwater CJ, Neil MJ. (1995). Optimal timing of wound drain removal following total joint arthroplasty. *J Arthroplasty*, Vol. 10, No. 2, (April 1995), pp. 185-189, ISSN 0883-5403

Ekbäck G, Axelsson K, Ryttberg L, Edlund B, Kjellberg J, Weckstrom J et al. (2000). Tranexamic acid reduces blood loss in total hip replacement surgery. *Anest Analg*, Vol. 91, No. 5, (November 2000), pp. 1124-1130, ISSN 0003-2999

Erceg M, Becić K. (2008). Postoperative closed suction drainage following hip and knee aloarthroplasty: drain removal after 24 or after 48 hours? *Lijec Vjesn*, Vol. 130, No. 5-6, (May-June 2008), pp. 133-135, ISSN 0024-3477

Johansson T, Engquist M, Pettersson LG, Lisander B. (2005). Blood loss after total hip replacement: a prospective randomized study between wound compression and drainage. *J Arthroplasty*, Vol. 20, No. 8, (December 2005), pp. 967-971, ISSN 0883-5403

Kim YH, Cho SH, Kim RS. (1998). Drainage versus nondrainage in simultaneous bilateral total hip arthroplasties. *J Arthroplasty*, Vol. 13, No. 2, (February 1998), pp. 156-161, ISSN 0883-5403

Kumar S, Penematsa S, Parekh S. (2007). Are drains required following a routine primary total joint arthroplasty? *Int Orthop*, Vol. 31, No. 5, (October 2007), pp. 593-596, ISSN 0341-2695

Levy, M. (1984). Intraperitoneal drainage. *Am J Surg*, Vol. 147, No. 3, (March 1984), pp. 309-314, ISSN 0002-9610

Murphy JP, Scott JE. (1993). The effectiveness od suction drainage in total hip arthroplasty. *J R Soc Med*, Vol. 86, No. 7, (July 1993), pp. 388-389, ISSN 0141-0768

Niskanen RO, Korkala OL, Haapala J, Kuokkanen HO, Kaukonen JP, Salo SA. (2000). Drainage is of no use in primary uncomplicated cemented hip and knee arthroplasty for osteoarthritis. A prospective randomized study. *J Arthroplasty*, Vol. 15, No. 5, (August 2000), pp. 567-569, ISSN 0883-5403

Ovadia D, Luger E, Menachem A, Dekel S. (1997). Efficacy of closed wound drainage after total joint arthroplasty. A prospective randomized study. *J Arthroplasty*, Vol. 12, No. 3, (April 1997), pp. 317-321, ISSN 0883-5403

Overgaard S, Thomsen NB, Kulinski B, Mossing NB. (1993). Closed suction drainage after hip arthroplasty. Prospective study of bacterial contamination in 81 cases. *Acta Orthop Scand*, Vol. 64, No. 4, (August 1993), pp. 417-420, ISSN 0001-6470

Parrini L, Baratelli M, Parrini M. (1988). Ultrasound examination of haematomas after total hip replacement. *Int Orthop*, Vol. 12, No. 1, pp. 79-82, ISSN 0341-2695

Parvizi J, Ghanem E, Joshi A, Sharkey PF, Hozack WJ, Rothman RH. (2007). Does "excessive" anticoagulation predispose to periprosthetic infection? *J Arthroplasty*, Vol. 22, No. 6 Suppl 2, (September 2007), pp. 24-28, ISSN 0883-5403

Patel VP, Walsh M, Sehgal B, Preston C, DeWal H, Cesare PE. (2007). Factors associated with prolonged wound drainage after primary total hip and knee arthroplasty. *J Bone Joint Surg Am*, Vol. 89, No. 1, (January 2007), pp. 33-38, ISSN 0021-9355

Ritter MA, Keating M, Faris PM. (1994). Closed wound drainage in total hip or total knee replacement. A prospective, randomized study. *J Bone J Surg Am*, Vol. 76, No. 1, (January 1994), pp. 35-38, ISSN 0021-9355

Rowe SM, Yoon TR, Kim YS, Lee GH. (1993). Hemovac drainage after hip arthroplasty. *Int Orthop*, Vol. 17, No. 4, pp. 238-240, ISSN 0341-2695

Saleh K, Olson M, Resig S, Bershadsky B, Kuskowski M, Gioe T, et al. (2002). Predictors of wound infection in hip and knee joint replacement: results from a 20 year surveillance program. *J Orthop Res*, Vol. 20, No. 3, (May 2002), pp. 506-515, ISSN 0736-0266

Singh J, Ballal MS, Mitchell P, Denn PG. (2010). Effects of tranexamic acid on blood loss during total hip arthroplasty. *J Orthop* Surg (Hong Kong), Vol. 18, No. 3, (December 2010), pp. 282-286, ISSN 1022-5536

Sørensen AI, Sørensen TS. (1991). Bacterial growth on suction drain tips. *Acta Orthop Scand*, Vol. 62, No. 5, (October 1991), pp. 451-454, ISSN 0001-6470

Strahovnik A, Fokter SK, Kotnik M. (2010). Comparison of drainage techniques on prolonged serous drainage after total hip arthroplasty. *J Arthroplasty*, Vol. 25, No. 2, (February 2010), pp. 244-248, ISSN 0883-5403

Walmsley PJ, Kelly MB, Hill RF, Brenkel I. (2005). A prospective, randomised, controlled trial of the use o drains in total hip arthroplasty. *J Bone J Surg Br*, Vol. 87, No. 10, (October 2005), pp. 1397-1401, ISSN 0301-620X

Waugh TR, Stinchfield FE. (1961). Suction drainage of orthopaedic wounds. *J Bone Joint Surg Am*, Vol. 43, (October 1961), pp. 939-946, ISSN 0021-9355

Weber EW, Slappendel R, Prins MH, van der Schaaf DB, Durieux ME, Strumper D. (2005). Perioperative blood transfusions and delayed wound healing after hip replacement surgery: Effects on duration of hospitalization. *Anesth Analg*, Vol. 100, No. 5, (May 2005), pp. 1416-1421, ISSN 0003-2999

Widman J, Jacobsson H, Larsson SA, Isacson J. (2002). No effect of drains on the postoperative hematoma volume in hip replacement surgery. A randomized study using scintigraphy. *Acta Orthop Scand*, Vol. 73, No. 6, (December 2002), pp. 625-629, ISSN 0001-6470

Willett KM, Simmons CD, Bentley G. (1988). The effect of suction drains after total hip replacement. *J Bone Joint Surg Br*, Vol. 70. No. 4, (August 1988), pp. 607-610, ISSN 0301-620X

Wood JJ, Bevis PM, Bannister GC. (2007). Wound oozing after total hip arthroplasty. *Ann R Coll Surg Eng*, Vol. 89, No. 2, (March 2007), pp. 140-142, ISSN 0035-8843

7

Methods for Optimising Patient Function After Total Hip Arthroplasty

Tosan Okoro[1,2], Andrew Lemmey[1],
Peter Maddison[1,2] and John G. Andrew[2]
[1]Bangor University,
[2]Ysbyty Gwynedd, Betsi Cadwaladr
University Health Board, Bangor
United Kingdom

1. Introduction

Symptomatic hip osteoarthritis occurs in 3% of the elderly (Felson 2004) and is associated with poor general health status (Dawson et al. 2004). Treatment strategies for hip pain have traditionally involved conservative measures (analgesia, exercise, education, weight reduction) and surgical intervention (joint replacement) is the most effective treatment for end stage disease (Birrell et al. 2000, Di Domenica et al. 2005).

According to the National joint registry, the number of primary total hip replacements (THR) in England and Wales in 2008/2009 totalled 77608, which is a steady rise from the amount reported in 2007/2008 (73632) and 2006/2007 (51981) (National Joint Registry for England and Wales 2010). The average age of patients undergoing a primary total hip replacement is 66.7 years (SD 13.1) with females slightly older than males (average 68.4 years (SD12.4) vs. 65.8 years (SD 12.24) respectively) (National Joint Registry for England and Wales 2010).

As technology and surgical techniques for total hip replacement (THR) improve, patient expectations have also increased, including for an early return to normal physical function and activities (Wang, Gilbey & Ackland 2002). A reduced time between surgery and mobilisation has been found to have an influence in reducing length of stay and increasing patient satisfaction (Husted et al. 2008). This is particularly important due to the introduction of initiatives such as integrated care pathways, which have rapidly reduced the length of hospital stay following joint replacement with inpatient physiotherapy time also reduced (National Audit Office 2003). The median length of stay for THR patients according to data collated from a total of 125 acute trusts in England (2004-2005) was 7 days (interquartile range IQR 5-10) (Wilson et al. 2008).

Whilst THR generally resolves pain, function usually remains substantially sub-optimal. At 24 months following total joint arthroplasty, patients with low pre-operative function are five times more likely to require assistance from another person for their activities of daily living compared to those with high preoperative function (relative risk 5.2, 95% CI 1.9-14.6; (Fortin et al. 2002)). This protracted disability has detrimental economic, social and health consequences. Optimising function after surgery is therefore an important component of rehabilitation.

2. Predictors of outcome following total hip replacement

A recent prospective multivariate regression analysis of factors affecting outcome after THR has shown that the most important factor to influence outcome is the preoperative Western Ontario and McMaster Universities Osteoarthritis (WOMAC) physical function (PF) score (Wang et al. 2009). WOMAC is one of the most widely used disease-specific outcome instruments in people with osteoarthritis. The study by Wang et al identified three independent variables; pre-operative WOMAC PF score, gender and the presence of co morbidities as significantly affecting the WOMAC PF score at 1 year post-operatively. Previous studies have hypothesised that high preoperative functional status has a positive effect on outcome whilst others have suggested that it leaves little room for improvement in functional status (Montin et al. 2008, Roder et al. 2007, Young et al. 1998). Patients with better preoperative functional scores are likely to have higher postoperative scores, whereas patients with poorer preoperative scores are likely to experience greater improvements in function (Wang et al. 2009). Greater improvement in functional outcome are observed in male vs. female patients and this could be due to the fact that women are more likely than men to seek THR at the more advanced stages of their disease (Katz et al. 1994).

Patients with preoperative co morbidities are more likely to have a poorer short-term outcome in terms of physical function and this recent finding by Wang et al is consistent in the literature (Lubbeke et al. 2007, Roder et al. 2003, Wood, McLauchlan 2006). Patients with significant preoperative co morbidities have more inpatient complications such as hypotension, neuropathy, thromboembolic events, septicaemia, cardiac arrest, myocardial infarction, respiratory failure, and renal failure after THR than those who do not (Imamura & Black 1998). Patients with hip osteoarthritis with musculoskeletal co morbidities such as low back pain and osteoarthritis of the non-operated hip, have less long term functional improvement after THR (Nilsdotter et al. 2003). A combination of more pain pre-operatively, higher age and postoperative low back pain predicts a worse outcome after THR in WOMAC PF after 3.6 years of follow-up (Nilsdotter et al. 2003). Function and pain in patients with lower preoperative physical function does not to improve postoperatively to the level achieved by those with higher preoperative function (Fortin et al. 1999).

Old age predicts a poor postoperative outcome after THR and this is consistent with the impression that older people with self reported conditions restricting mobility in addition to arthritic pain in the hip or knee are at higher risk of psychological distress and physical dysfunction (Nilsdotter et al. 2003, Hopman-Rock et al. 1997).

3. Muscle strength and its relation to function after total hip replacement

The most common preoperative complaints by patients who elect to have THR are pain and loss of mobility (Trudelle-Jackson, Smith 2004). It therefore follows that the most commonly reported outcomes of THR in the literature relate to pain relief and restoration of mobility (Trudelle-Jackson, Smith 2004). Outcome studies of pain reduction and range of motion restoration, usually conducted 3 to 6 months after THR, indicate an overall satisfaction by patients and physicians (Barber et al. 1996). Outcome studies performed at least 1 year after THR reveal that impairments and functional limitations persist in the absence of pain. Impairments that persist at least 1 year after THR include decreased muscle strength and postural stability on the side of the replaced hip (Trudelle-Jackson et al. 2002). There are reported deficits in muscle strength of the involved hip after THR of 10-21% when compared to the uninvolved hip at 1 year post-surgery (Trudelle-Jackson et al. 2002, Shih et al. 1994). The atrophic changes that occur about the hip persist up to 2 years following THR and this is evidenced by increased fat infiltration (Rasch et al. 2009). There is a suggestion by the authors that earlier operation may prevent the development of these changes and that fatty infiltration may be reversed by intensive rehabilitation (Rasch et al. 2009).

Frail elderly persons with sarcopenia (degenerative loss of skeletal muscle mass and strength associated with aging) often undergo musculoskeletal-related surgery, and the hospitalisation-associated immobilisation further compromises the skeletal system, with potentially grave consequences (Suetta et al. 2004). Many elderly patients fail to regain their preoperative level of function and self-care (Sashika et al. 1996).

Immobilisation due to major surgery and hospitalisation can cause a severe decline in muscle mass, muscle strength and muscle function (Bloomfield 1997, Covinsky et al. 2003, Hill et al. 1993). Muscle strength declines 4% per day during the first week of immobilisation, making it very important that physical training is commenced as soon as possible after surgery (Wigerstad-Lossing et al. 1988).

Physical training can improve strength and functional performance in healthy elderly and frail nursing home residents (Harridge et al. 1999, Lexell et al. 1995). Supervised progressive resistance training (PRT) in the early post-operative phase has been shown to be effective in restoring muscle mass, contractile rate of force development, and functional performance than rehabilitation regimes based on functional exercises and electrical stimulation (Suetta et al. 2004). Strength training that is initiated 6 to 8 weeks or more than 6 months after hip surgery also significantly increases muscle strength (Sashika et al. 1996, Hauer et al. 2002). Recent studies suggest this is feasible in a supervised facility and that it offers an effective way of increasing maximal muscle strength in elderly postoperative patients with significant gains in muscle fibre size and pennation angle that resemble those typically seen in young healthy individuals (Suetta et al. 2008).

Gait dysfunctions and asymmetries, both pre-and post-THR surgery, are also evident in patients with unilateral hip osteoarthritis (Madsen et al. 2004). This is inherently dangerous because it is well known that gait dysfunctions or lower limb muscular weakness heighten the risk of falls especially when negotiating uneven terrain such as a step or a chair (Madsen et al. 2004). Dysfunction can also lead to reduced mobility, living independence, and physical activity levels (Galea et al. 2008)

4. Impact of aging on muscle

Aging and disuse are two of the main conditions leading to skeletal muscle atrophy in humans (Suetta et al. 2008). In both conditions, the loss of muscle mass leads to a decrease in muscle force production, and there may also be a significant additional contribution from changes in muscle architecture (Narici et al, 2005). The loss of muscle mass with aging accelerates from the sixth decade onward, partly owing to a decreased number of muscle fibres and also as the result of general muscle fibre atrophy (Lexell et al, 1991). Cross sectional studies indicate that type II fibres are more vulnerable to the aging process than type I fibres (Lexell et al, 1991) but other studies have found more marked type I atrophy (Frontera et al, 2000). Muscle mass has been estimated to decrease by 30% during the life span (Lexell et al, 1995) and maximal muscle strength is reduced as a result of aging by~1.5% per year from the sixth decade onwards (Skelton et al. 1994). Muscle strength has also been shown to decrease approximately 50% from age 30 to 80 (Sinaki 2004). Marked alterations in muscle architecture potentially contribute to loss of muscle strength (Narici et al, 2005) and muscle fibre pennation angle reduction of 10-13% in old compared to young individuals suggests this (Narici et al, 2003).

5. Exercise regimes for improving function

One hour of physical training twice a week increases the muscle strength in the quadriceps muscle by 21% and grip strength by 14% with not more than eight weeks of physical training (Heislein et al, 1994). Similarly, low to moderate physical activity during 16 weeks of physical training is associated with a 30-100% increase in muscle strength in both men and women while the bone mass (BM) at best increases by 3% (Ryan et al. 1994). There are reports that muscle strength increases by up to 200% even in octogenarians, a much larger increase than the 2-20% increases in muscle volume or the 1-2% increases in BM with a similar training program (Daley & Spinks 2000, Fiatarone et al. 1994, Lexell 1999, Province et al. 1995).

Women above age 60 who exercise with aerobics twice per week improve their balance, co-ordination and muscle strength (Lord et al. 1995). The muscle strength in the quadriceps muscle improved by 29% and the sway of the body was reduced by 6%, while the BM was unchanged during the intervention year. The most commonly used rehabilitation regimes for elderly individuals are based on functional types of exercises without external loading (Suetta et al. 2008), although this type of intervention does not prevent further muscle atrophy (Reardon et al. 2001). Resistance training is an effective method to induce muscle hypertrophy and increase muscle strength and functional performance in the elderly (Harridge et al 1999) and using it in the postoperative phase has been shown to be an effective method to restore muscle function in this group of patients (Hauer et al. 2002).

Progressive resistance training (PRT) by definition elicits positive health and performance adaptations by challenging the skeletal muscles with loads that can be lifted repetitively to the onset of neuromuscular fatigue, the point at which appropriate technique can no longer be maintained (American College of Sports Medicine, 1998). PRT sessions are optimal when followed by periods of recovery ranging from 48 to 72 h to allow for physiological super compensation (i.e. positive adaptation) (Cheema et al. 2007). To facilitate continued adaptation, training intensity (i.e. load) and volume (i.e. number of sets) are progressively increased, and exercises are adjusted as indicated throughout the training regimen, to attenuate the onset of a plateau in physiological adaptation. Once the physiological plateau has been reached, health and performance are maintained with continued training, which may involve periodical manipulations of the PRT variables, including training frequency, training intensity (load), training volume (sets), types of exercises, and time under tension per repetition (Cheema et al. 2007).

PRT is a well-established and safe exercise modality for individuals of all ages and fitness levels, including those afflicted with severe chronic illnesses (Fiatarone et al. 1994, Cheema et al. 2007). It is particularly efficacious for adult and elderly cohorts given its efficacy in counteracting sarcopenia, abating osteoporosis and helping reverse the physiological and functional impairments that accrue with age (Fiatarone et al. 1994).

6. The evidence for pre-operative exercise regimes

Appropriate exercise offers many benefits in treating the patient with osteoarthritis (Macera et al. 2003). Stronger, better-conditioned periarticular muscles, tendons, and ligaments have advantageous biomechanical effects on attenuating joint forces during movement (Felson et al. 2000). In more severe disease, which often leads to reduced mobility and disuse atrophy, exercise can improve pain, muscle strength, cardiovascular fitness, self-efficacy, and function (van Baar et al. 1999).

Exercise is a cornerstone of rehabilitation following total joint arthroplasty and other surgical procedures (Eyigor et al. 2004). Using exercise in the pre-operative period has variable benefit. An improvement has been demonstrated in the preoperative functional status after a 6 week presurgical exercise program (water and land based strength training activities) in patients awaiting total hip and knee arthroplasty in comparison to patients having routine rehabilitation but this effect is not maintained after 8 and 26 weeks of follow up (Rooks et al. 2006). This fits in with a previous study by Wijgman et al (Wijgman et al. 1994), which reported that preoperative physical therapy and instruction were not useful for patients before total hip arthoplasty. In their sample of 31 patients, few differences were observed between the patients and control subjects on measures such as the visual analogue pain scale and the Harris hip score (Wijgman et al. 1994). More recent work by Gocen et al (Gocen et al. 2004) also showed that instruction and pre-operative physiotherapy is of no benefit in terms of improving outcome (measured with the Harris Hip Score and Visual analogue scale) after THR surgery.

A systematic review by Ackerman and Bennell (Ackerman & Bennell 2004) found that only two randomised controlled trials involving patients undergoing THR surgery demonstrated a benefit of performing pre-operative exercise. Both Wang et al (Wang, Gilbey & Ackland 2002) and Gilbey et al (Gilbey et al. 2003) used pre-operative stationary bikes, resistance training of the lower limb and hydrotherapy with post-operative hydrotherapy, progressive strengthening exercises and aerobic activity. Wang et al (Wang, Gilbey & Ackland 2002) reported a significantly higher mean gait velocity for the exercise group from three to 24 weeks post-operatively, and a greater mean distance walked by the exercise group at 24 weeks post-operatively. Gilbey et al (Gilbey et al. 2003) found that the exercise group experienced significantly larger gains in hip strength, WOMAC scores, and hip ROM from three to 24 weeks post-operatively. The systematic review concluded that the major limitation of these studies was the addition of an intensive post-operative exercise program for the intervention group only, so it is impossible to determine which of the pre-operative regimes was responsible for the improvements seen. There is therefore a lack of conclusive evidence to justify the use of pre-operative regimes to optimise function after THR surgery.

7. The evidence for post-operative home or centre-based exercise regimes to improve function

Early targeted rehabilitation has been shown to reduce hospital length of stay without an increase in complication rates after THR (Iyengar et al. 2007). Exercise programs beyond the normal postoperative rehabilitation period have been shown to reduce pain and leg stiffness, improve physical function and lessen the chance of accidental falls in THR patients (Gilbey et al. 2003). A disadvantage of these programs is the need for patients to exercise under the supervision of professional staff at a hospital or rehabilitation centre (Galea et al. 2008). This makes program delivery expensive due to the high costs associated with supervision, treatment and transport (Galea et al. 2008). In addition, some THR patients are excluded because difficulties with mobility and transport to a centre exclude participation (Marottoli et al, 1992). Studies comparing home- and centre-based rehabilitation programs for THR patients have found no difference in WOMAC scores, complication rates and patient satisfaction after 3 and 12 months of follow up (Mahomed et al. 2008).

An important factor in both home and centre based regimes is the use of PRT. A systematic review performed by the author (manuscript submitted for publication) on level 1 evidence-(randomised controlled trials) for regimes for rehabilitation after THR found the use of PRT to be predictive of functional benefit, when measured either using objective measures such as muscle strength or subjective functional measures such as the WOMAC. These centre-based interventions (Hesse et al, 2003; Husby et al, 2009; Jesudason et al, 2002; Liebs et al, 2010; Suetta et al, 2004) were performed in the early period (<1 month following surgery) and the home-based interventions (Jan et al, 2004; Trudelle-Jackson et al 2004) were performed late (>1 month following surgery).

A limitation of the home-based interventions assessed in the literature is that follow-up does not extend beyond the end of the exercise interventions periods. Thus, it is not clear whether the benefits evident at the end of the exercise intervention are maintained in the longer term. The other obvious shortcoming is the lateness of the intervention in the home setting and consequently the failure to ameliorate or prevent the exacerbated loss of muscle and function after surgery. A recent systematic review by Di Monaco et al (Di Monaco et al. 2009) suggests that the difficulties in THR rehabilitation research are that there is a lack of multicentre clinical trials with large sample sizes to inform the design of optimal physical exercise programs.

8. Motivators and barriers to improving function through exercise

Routine physical exercise improves one's general physical health (Wang et al. 2002) decreases the risk of medical conditions such as coronary artery disease, diabetes, osteoporosis and hypertension (Bouchard & Despres 1995); reduces mental health concerns such as depression (Newson & Kemps 2007); and can prevent falls (Barnett et al. 2003). Recent research also suggests that physical exercise plays a role in the maintenance of cognitive vitality in older age (Colcombe et al. 2004).

A recent study has shown that specific motivators and barriers to exercise differ with age, education, gender, psychological and physical well-being and current level of exercise (Newson & Kemps 2007). People over the age of 75 are more likely to be motivated to exercise purely to maintain an active lifestyle than those aged 63 to 74 years, and medical problems are more likely to prevent them from engaging in exercise compared than their younger counterparts (Newson & Kemps 2007). Men were found to be more likely than women to be motivated to exercise for the challenging nature of exercise. On the other hand, women are more likely than men to report health concerns as a reason to exercise, and they are more likely to blame a lack of exercise facilities and exercise specific knowledge as factors to prevent them from exercising (Newson & Kemps 2007).

High-level exercisers find the challenge to exercise to be more of a motivator than their low level counterparts, who reported health concerns to be a more important motivator. Low-level exercisers also noted a concern that factors associated with exercise and a lack of facilities and knowledge about exercise prevented them from exercising (Newson & Kemps 2007). The authors conclude that intervention programs for older adults need to take into account the specific contextual factors of the individual. The average age of patients undergoing THR surgery in the UK is 66.7 years (National Joint Registry for England and Wales 2010). According to Newson et al, these patients (63-74 years old) view keeping their fitness (feel-good nature of exercise, enjoyment) as the most important motivator whilst the most significant barrier is situational i.e. having no one to exercise with, disliking exercising alone and adverse weather conditions.

9. Outcome measures for assessing function

The need for THR is predicted to grow by 174% between 2005 and 2030 (Kurtz et al. 2007). It is therefore important that patient outcomes after surgery are continuously monitored and reviewed, to improve practise and optimise outcomes after surgery (Wylde et al. 2009). Central to assessing the effectiveness of hip replacement in a clinical setting is choosing the appropriate outcome measure (Wylde et al. 2009). In orthopaedics, outcomes after surgery can be assessed using five different methods, namely radiographic analysis, implant survivorship analysis, surgeon-based outcome measures, performance-related assessment and patient reported outcome questionnaires (Wylde et al. 2009).

Performance related assessment involves assessing the individual as they perform a specific task that is evaluated in a standardised manner using predetermined criteria (Wylde et al. 2009). A recent review (Terwee et al. 2006) has found that 26 performance measures have been used to assess function in patients with lower limb arthritis or joint replacement including walking, stair-climbing and chair tests. A moderate correlation has been reported between the results of patient self-reported functional ability and performance measures (Stratford et al. 2003; Terwee et al. 2006). This could be because performance related tests may not reflect the true demands and exertions associated with activities of daily living (Wylde et al. 2009). Other limitations include the fact that they are time consuming and only consider physical function whilst neglecting other important domains of outcome such as pain, quality of life and general well-being (Terwee et al. 2006).

Generic Health	Disease specific	Joint-specific
Assess subjective general health status with comparisons across different disease states and treatment options	Focus solely on symptom and disabilities relating to particular condition but are not particular to the joint of assessment.	Specific to the joint of assessment and attempt to exclude the influence of co morbidities
e.g. SF36. Assesses 8 dimensions of health related quality of life (HRQoL): Bodily pain, physical role functioning, physical role limitations, general health, vitality, social role functioning, emotional role limitations and mental health.	e.g. for Rheumatoid arthritis AIMS (Arthritis Impact Measurement Scale) which has 9 component scales which assess mobility, physical activity, social activity, social role, activities of daily living, pain, dexterity, anxiety and depression. For Osteoarthritis, Western Ontario and McMaster University Osteoarthritis index (WOMAC) which is a 24 item measure of pain, stiffness and function.	E.g. Oxford Hip score which is a short 12 item questionnaire specifically developed to assess functional ability and pain in patients undergoing hip replacement. The questionnaire displays good psychometric properties and has a larger effect size than other tools such as the SF36.

Table 1. Types of Patient Reported Outcome Measures (PROMs) (Bellamy et al. 1988; Brazier et al. 1992; Dawson et al. 1998; Jenkinson & Layte 1997; Meenan et al. 1980; Salaffi et al. 2005; Ware et al. 1992, 1996)

Surgeon based assessment tools such as the Harris Hip Score assume concordance between the view of patients and clinicians, which is an erroneous assumption across all healthcare settings (Wylde et al. 2009). Within Orthopaedics, a lack of correlation has been demonstrated between surgeon and patient ratings of pain, function and satisfaction after joint replacement (Anderson et al. 1996; Bullens et al. 2001).Whereas surgeons may judge the success of joint replacement on the range of motion, alignment and stability, patients may evaluate outcome in terms of vitality and ability to return to leisure activities (Wylde et al. 2009). This inconsistency between patient and clinician ratings of health has guided the development of rigorous validated patient-reported outcome measures (Wylde et al. 2009).

Patient reported outcome measures (PROMs) are advantageous because they are a cost-effective, efficient and minimally intrusive method of collecting data on patients (Wylde et al. 2009). PROMS can be grouped into generic health, disease specific and joint specific (Table 1). A limitation of all PROMs is the issue of recall bias towards patients reporting the most severe and recent pain they have experienced (Jensen et al. 2008).

10. Areas that remain to be explored

Total hip replacement surgery provides good relief for patients' pain but fails to fully restore physical function. The impairment of muscle function that occurs in relation to aging is exacerbated by the impact of surgery and subsequent immobilisation. Pre-operative regimes to improve functional outcome have not been shown to be beneficial. Post-operative regimes on the other hand, if including PRT, appear to have a significant benefit on patient function following THR regardless of the timing of the intervention. Centre-based regimes are plagued with issues of high transport and supervision costs. Early home based PRT studies that are effective and safe; with adequate follow-up after THR surgery would potentially improve outcomes after THR at an affordable cost, and appear an important area for future research.

11. Acknowledgements

I would like to dedicate this chapter to Iyé, Roli and Edosa- the rocks on which I build my world. I would also like to thank the North Wales Research Committee for their support.

12. References

"American College of Sports Medicine Position Stand. The recommended quantity and quality of exercise for developing and maintaining cardiorespiratory and muscular fitness, and flexibility in healthy adults", 1998, Medicine and science in sports and exercise, vol. 30, no. 6, pp. 975-991.

Ackerman, I.N. & Bennell, K.L. 2004, "Does pre-operative physiotherapy improve outcomes from lower limb joint replacement surgery? A systematic review", The Australian journal of physiotherapy, vol. 50, no. 1, pp. 25-30.

Anderson, J.G., Wixson, R.L., Tsai, D., Stulberg, S.D. & Chang, R.W. 1996, "Functional outcome and patient satisfaction in total knee patients over the age of 75", The Journal of arthroplasty, vol. 11, no. 7, pp. 831-840.

Barber, T.C., Roger, D.J., Goodman, S.B. & Schurman, D.J. 1996, "Early outcome of total hip arthroplasty using the direct
lateral vs the posterior surgical approach", Orthopedics, vol. 19, no. 10, pp. 873-875.

Barnett, A., Smith, B., Lord, S.R., Williams, M. & Baumand, A. 2003, "Community-based group exercise improves balance and reduces falls in at-risk older people: a randomised controlled trial", Age and Ageing, vol. 32, no. 4, pp. 407-414.

Bellamy, N., Buchanan, W.W., Goldsmith, C.H., Campbell, J. & Stitt, L.W. 1988, "Validation study of WOMAC: a health status instrument for measuring clinically important patient relevant outcomes to antirheumatic drug therapy in patients with osteoarthritis of the hip or knee", The Journal of rheumatology, vol. 15, no. 12, pp. 1833-1840.

Birrell, F., Croft, P., Cooper, C., Hosie, G., Macfarlane, G.J. & Silman, A. 2000, "Radiographic change is common in new presenters in primary care with hip pain. PCR Hip Study Group", Rheumatology (Oxford, England), vol. 39, no. 7, pp. 772-775.

Bloomfield, S.A. 1997, "Changes in musculoskeletal structure and function with prolonged bed rest", Medicine and science in sports and exercise, vol. 29, no. 2, pp. 197-206.

Bouchard, C. & Despres, J.P. 1995, "Physical activity and health: atherosclerotic, metabolic, and hypertensive diseases", Research quarterly for exercise and sport, vol. 66, no. 4, pp. 268-275.

Bullens, P.H., van Loon, C.J., de Waal Malefijt, M.C., Laan, R.F. & Veth, R.P. 2001, "Patient satisfaction after total knee arthroplasty: a comparison between subjective and objective outcome assessments", The Journal of arthroplasty, vol. 16, no. 6, pp. 740-747.

Cheema, B., Abas, H., Smith, B., O'Sullivan, A., Chan, M., Patwardhan, A., Kelly, J., Gillin, A., Pang, G., Lloyd, B. & Singh, M.F. 2007, "Progressive exercise for anabolism in kidney disease (PEAK): a randomized, controlled trial of resistance training during hemodialysis", Journal of the American Society of Nephrology : JASN, vol. 18, no. 5, pp. 1594-1601.

Colcombe, S.J., Kramer, A.F., McAuley, E., Erickson, K.I. & Scalf, P. 2004, "Neurocognitive aging and cardiovascular fitness: recent findings and future directions", Journal of molecular neuroscience : MN, vol. 24, no. 1, pp. 9-14.

Covinsky, K.E., Palmer, R.M., Fortinsky, R.H., Counsell, S.R., Stewart, A.L., Kresevic, D., Burant, C.J. & Landefeld, C.S. 2003, "Loss of independence in activities of daily living in older adults hospitalized with medical illnesses: increased vulnerability with age", Journal of the American Geriatrics Society, vol. 51, no. 4, pp. 451-458.

Daley, M.J. & Spinks, W.L. 2000, "Exercise, mobility and aging", Sports medicine (Auckland, N.Z.), vol. 29, no. 1, pp. 1-12.

Dawson, J., Fitzpatrick, R., Murray, D. & Carr, A. 1998, "Questionnaire on the perceptions of patients about total knee replacement", The Journal of bone and joint surgery.British volume, vol. 80, no. 1, pp. 63-69.

Dawson, J., Linsell, L., Zondervan, K., Rose, P., Randall, T., Carr, A. & Fitzpatrick, R. 2004, "Epidemiology of hip and knee pain and its impact on overall health status in older adults", Rheumatology (Oxford, England), vol. 43, no. 4, pp. 497-504.

Di Domenica, F., Sarzi-Puttini, P., Cazzola, M., Atzeni, F., Cappadonia, C., Caserta, A., Galletti, R., Volonte, L. & Mele, G. 2005, "Physical and rehabilitative approaches in osteoarthritis", Seminars in arthritis and rheumatism, vol. 34, no. 6 Suppl 2, pp. 62-69.

Di Monaco, M., Vallero, F., Tappero, R. & Cavanna, A. 2009, "Rehabilitation after total hip arthroplasty: a systematic review of controlled trials on physical exercise programs", European journal of physical and rehabilitation medicine, vol. 45, no. 3, pp. 303-317.

Eyigor, S., Hepguler, S. & Capaci, K. 2004, "A comparison of muscle training methods in patients with knee osteoarthritis", Clinical rheumatology, vol. 23, no. 2, pp. 109-115.

Felson, D.T., Lawrence, R.C., Dieppe, P.A., Hirsch, R., Helmick, C.G., Jordan, J.M., Kington, R.S., Lane, N.E., Nevitt, M.C., Zhang, Y., Sowers, M., McAlindon, T., Spector, T.D., Poole, A.R., Yanovski, S.Z., Ateshian, G., Sharma, L., Buckwalter, J.A., Brandt, K.D. & Fries, J.F. 2000, "Osteoarthritis: new insights. Part 1: the disease and its risk factors", Annals of Internal Medicine, vol. 133, no. 8, pp. 635-646.

Fiatarone, M.A., O'Neill, E.F., Ryan, N.D., Clements, K.M., Solares, G.R., Nelson, M.E., Roberts, S.B., Kehayias, J.J., Lipsitz, L.A. & Evans, W.J. 1994, "Exercise training and nutritional supplementation for physical frailty in very elderly people", The New England journal of medicine, vol. 330, no. 25, pp. 1769-1775.

Fortin, P.R., Clarke, A.E., Joseph, L., Liang, M.H., Tanzer, M., Ferland, D., Phillips, C., Partridge, A.J., Belisle, P., Fossel, A.H., Mahomed, N., Sledge, C.B. & Katz, J.N. 1999, "Outcomes of total hip and knee replacement: preoperative functional status predicts outcomes at six months after surgery", Arthritis and Rheumatism, vol. 42, no. 8, pp. 1722-1728.

Fortin, P.R., Penrod, J.R., Clarke, A.E., St-Pierre, Y., Joseph, L., Belisle, P., Liang, M.H., Ferland, D., Phillips, C.B., Mahomed, N., Tanzer, M., Sledge, C., Fossel, A.H. & Katz, J.N. 2002, "Timing of total joint replacement affects clinical outcomes among patients with osteoarthritis of the hip or knee", Arthritis and Rheumatism, vol. 46, no. 12, pp. 3327-3330.

Frontera, W.R., Hughes, V.A., Fielding, R.A., Fiatarone, M.A., Evans, W.J. & Roubenoff, R. 2000, "Aging of skeletal muscle: a 12-yr longitudinal study", Journal of applied physiology (Bethesda, Md.: 1985), vol. 88, no. 4, pp. 1321-1326.

Galea, M.P., Levinger, P., Lythgo, N., Cimoli, C., Weller, R., Tully, E., McMeeken, J. & Westh, R. 2008, "A targeted home- and center-based exercise program for people after total hip replacement: a randomized clinical trial", Archives of Physical Medicine and Rehabilitation, vol. 89, no. 8, pp. 1442-1447.

Gilbey, H.J., Ackland, T.R., Wang, A.W., Morton, A.R., Trouchet, T. & Tapper, J. 2003, "Exercise improves early functional recovery after total hip arthroplasty", Clinical orthopaedics and related research, vol. (408), no. 408, pp. 193-200.

Gocen, Z., Sen, A., Unver, B., Karatosun, V. & Gunal, I. 2004, "The effect of preoperative physiotherapy and education on the outcome of total hip replacement: a prospective randomized controlled trial", Clinical rehabilitation, vol. 18, no. 4, pp. 353-358.

Harridge, S.D., Kryger, A. & Stensgaard, A. 1999, "Knee extensor strength, activation, and size in very elderly people following strength training", Muscle & nerve, vol. 22, no. 7, pp. 831-839.

Hauer, K., Specht, N., Schuler, M., Bartsch, P. & Oster, P. 2002, "Intensive physical training in geriatric patients after severe falls and hip surgery", Age and Ageing, vol. 31, no. 1, pp. 49-57.

Heislein, D.M., Harris, B.A. & Jette, A.M. 1994, "A strength training program for postmenopausal women: a pilot study", Archives of Physical Medicine and Rehabilitation, vol. 75, no. 2, pp. 198-204.

Hesse, S., Werner, C., Seibel, H., von Frankenberg, S., Kappel, E.M., Kirker, S. & Kading, M. 2003, "Treadmill training with partial body-weight support after total hip arthroplasty: a randomized controlled trial", Archives of Physical Medicine and Rehabilitation, vol. 84, no. 12, pp. 1767-1773.

Hill, G.L., Douglas, R.G. & Schroeder, D. 1993, "Metabolic basis for the management of patients undergoing major surgery", World journal of surgery, vol. 17, no. 2, pp. 146-153.

Hopman-Rock, M., Odding, E., Hofman, A., Kraaimaat, F.W. & Bijlsma, J.W. 1997, "Differences in health status of older adults with pain in the hip or knee only and with additional mobility restricting conditions", The Journal of rheumatology, vol. 24, no. 12, pp. 2416-2423.

Husby, V.S., Helgerud, J., Bjorgen, S., Husby, O.S., Benum, P. & Hoff, J. 2009, "Early maximal strength training is an efficient treatment for patients operated with total hip arthroplasty", Archives of Physical Medicine and Rehabilitation, vol. 90, no. 10, pp. 1658-1667.

Husted, H., Holm, G. & Jacobsen, S. 2008, "Predictors of length of stay and patient satisfaction after hip and knee replacement surgery: fast-track experience in 712 patients", Acta orthopaedica, vol. 79, no. 2, pp. 168-173.

Imamura, K. & Black, N. 1998, "Does comorbidity affect the outcome of surgery? Total hip replacement in the UK and Japan", International journal for quality in health care : journal of the International Society for Quality in Health Care / ISQua, vol. 10, no. 2, pp. 113-123.

Iyengar, K.P., Nadkarni, J.B., Ivanovic, N. & Mahale, A. 2007, "Targeted early rehabilitation at home after total hip and knee joint replacement: Does it work?", Disability and rehabilitation, vol. 29, no. 6, pp. 495-502.

Jan, M.H., Hung, J.Y., Lin, J.C., Wang, S.F., Liu, T.K. & Tang, P.F. 2004, "Effects of a home program on strength, walking speed, and function after total hip replacement", Archives of Physical Medicine and Rehabilitation, vol. 85, no. 12, pp. 1943-1951.

Jenkinson, C. & Layte, R. 1997, "Development and testing of the UK SF-12 (short form health survey)", Journal of health services research & policy, vol. 2, no. 1, pp. 14-18.

Jesudason, C. & Stiller, K. 2002, "Are bed exercises necessary following hip arthroplasty?", The Australian journal of physiotherapy, vol. 48, no. 2, pp. 73-81.

Katz, J.N., Wright, E.A., Guadagnoli, E., Liang, M.H., Karlson, E.W. & Cleary, P.D. 1994, "Differences between men and women undergoing major orthopedic surgery for degenerative arthritis", Arthritis and Rheumatism, vol. 37, no. 5, pp. 687-694.

Kurtz, S., Ong, K., Lau, E., Mowat, F. & Halpern, M. 2007, "Projections of primary and revision hip and knee arthroplasty in the United States from 2005 to 2030", The Journal of bone and joint surgery.American volume, vol. 89, no. 4, pp. 780-785.

Lexell, J. 1999, "Effects of strength and endurance training on skeletal muscles in the elderly. New muscles for old!", Lakartidningen, vol. 96, no. 3, pp. 207-209.

Lexell, J. 1995, "Human aging, muscle mass, and fiber type composition", The journals of gerontology.Series A, Biological sciences and medical sciences, vol. 50 Spec No, pp. 11-16.

Lexell, J., Downham, D.Y., Larsson, Y., Bruhn, E. & Morsing, B. 1995, "Heavy-resistance training in older Scandinavian men and women: short- and long-term effects on arm and leg muscles", Scandinavian journal of medicine & science in sports, vol. 5, no. 6, pp. 329-341.

Lexell, J. & Taylor, C.C. 1991, "Variability in muscle fibre areas in whole human quadriceps muscle: effects of increasing age", Journal of anatomy, vol. 174, pp. 239-249.

Liebs, T.R., Herzberg, W., Ruther, W., Haasters, J., Russlies, M. & Hassenpflug, J. 2010, "Ergometer cycling after hip or knee replacement surgery: a randomized controlled trial", The Journal of bone and joint surgery.American volume, vol. 92, no. 4, pp. 814-822.

Lord, S.R., Ward, J.A., Williams, P. & Strudwick, M. 1995, "The effect of a 12-month exercise trial on balance, strength, and falls in older women: a randomized controlled trial", Journal of the American Geriatrics Society, vol. 43, no. 11, pp. 1198-1206.

Lubbeke, A., Katz, J.N., Perneger, T.V. & Hoffmeyer, P. 2007, "Primary and revision hip arthroplasty: 5-year outcomes and influence of age and comorbidity", The Journal of rheumatology, vol. 34, no. 2, pp. 394-400.

Macera, C.A., Hootman, J.M. & Sniezek, J.E. 2003, "Major public health benefits of physical activity", Arthritis and Rheumatism, vol. 49, no. 1, pp. 122-128.

Madsen, M.S., Ritter, M.A., Morris, H.H., Meding, J.B., Berend, M.E., Faris, P.M. & Vardaxis, V.G. 2004, "The effect of total hip arthroplasty surgical approach on gait", Journal of orthopaedic research : official publication of the Orthopaedic Research Society, vol. 22, no. 1, pp. 44-50.

Mahomed, N.N., Davis, A.M., Hawker, G., Badley, E., Davey, J.R., Syed, K.A., Coyte, P.C., Gandhi, R. & Wright, J.G. 2008, "Inpatient compared with home-based rehabilitation following primary unilateral total hip or knee replacement: a randomized controlled trial", The Journal of bone and joint surgery.American volume, vol. 90, no. 8, pp. 1673-1680.

Marottoli, R.A., Berkman, L.F. & Cooney, L.M.,Jr 1992, "Decline in physical function following hip fracture", Journal of the American Geriatrics Society, vol. 40, no. 9, pp. 861-866.

Meenan, R.F., Gertman, P.M. & Mason, J.H. 1980, "Measuring health status in arthritis. The arthritis impact measurement scales", Arthritis and Rheumatism, vol. 23, no. 2, pp. 146-152.

Montin, L., Leino-Kilpi, H., Suominen, T. & Lepisto, J. 2008, "A systematic review of empirical studies between 1966 and 2005 of patient outcomes of total hip arthroplasty and related factors", Journal of clinical nursing, vol. 17, no. 1, pp. 40-45.

Narici, M.V., Maganaris, C. & Reeves, N. 2005, "Myotendinous alterations and effects of resistive loading in old age", Scandinavian journal of medicine & science in sports, vol. 15, no. 6, pp. 392-401.

Narici, M.V., Maganaris, C.N., Reeves, N.D. & Capodaglio, P. 2003, "Effect of aging on human muscle architecture", Journal of applied physiology (Bethesda, Md.: 1985), vol. 95, no. 6, pp. 2229-2234.

National Audit Office 2003, Hip replacements: an update. HC 956.

National Joint Registry for England and Wales 2010, 7th Annual Clinical Report.

Newson, R.S. & Kemps, E.B. 2007, "Factors that promote and prevent exercise engagement in older adults", Journal of aging and health, vol. 19, no. 3, pp. 470-481.

Nilsdotter, A.K., Petersson, I.F., Roos, E.M. & Lohmander, L.S. 2003, "Predictors of patient relevant outcome after total hip replacement for osteoarthritis: a prospective study", Annals of the Rheumatic Diseases, vol. 62, no. 10, pp. 923-930.

Province, M.A., Hadley, E.C., Hornbrook, M.C., Lipsitz, L.A., Miller, J.P., Mulrow, C.D., Ory, M.G., Sattin, R.W., Tinetti, M.E. & Wolf, S.L. 1995, "The effects of exercise on falls in elderly patients. A preplanned meta-analysis of the FICSIT Trials. Frailty and Injuries: Cooperative Studies of Intervention Techniques", JAMA : the journal of the American Medical Association, vol. 273, no. 17, pp. 1341-1347.

Rasch, A., Bystrom, A.H., Dalen, N., Martinez-Carranza, N. & Berg, H.E. 2009, "Persisting muscle atrophy two years after replacement of the hip", The Journal of bone and joint surgery.British volume, vol. 91, no. 5, pp. 583-588.

Reardon, K., Galea, M., Dennett, X., Choong, P. & Byrne, E. 2001, "Quadriceps muscle wasting persists 5 months after total hip arthroplasty for osteoarthritis of the hip: a pilot study", Internal Medicine Journal, vol. 31, no. 1, pp. 7-14.

Roder, C., Parvizi, J., Eggli, S., Berry, D.J., Muller, M.E. & Busato, A. 2003, "Demographic factors affecting long-term outcome of total hip arthroplasty", Clinical orthopaedics and related research, vol. (417), no. 417, pp. 62-73.

Roder, C., Staub, L.P., Eggli, S., Dietrich, D., Busato, A. & Muller, U. 2007, "Influence of preoperative functional status on outcome after total hip arthroplasty", The Journal of bone and joint surgery.American volume, vol. 89, no. 1, pp. 11-17.

Rooks, D.S., Huang, J., Bierbaum, B.E., Bolus, S.A., Rubano, J., Connolly, C.E., Alpert, S., Iversen, M.D. & Katz, J.N. 2006, "Effect of preoperative exercise on measures of functional status in men and women undergoing total hip and knee arthroplasty", Arthritis and Rheumatism, vol. 55, no. 5, pp. 700-708.

Ryan, A.S., Treuth, M.S., Rubin, M.A., Miller, J.P., Nicklas, B.J., Landis, D.M., Pratley, R.E., Libanati, C.R., Gundberg, C.M. & Hurley, B.F. 1994, "Effects of strength training on bone mineral density: hormonal and bone turnover relationships", Journal of applied physiology (Bethesda, Md.: 1985), vol. 77, no. 4, pp. 1678-1684.

Salaffi, F., Carotti, M. & Grassi, W. 2005, "Health-related quality of life in patients with hip or knee osteoarthritis: comparison of generic and disease-specific instruments", Clinical rheumatology, vol. 24, no. 1, pp. 29-37.

Sashika, H., Matsuba, Y. & Watanabe, Y. 1996, "Home program of physical therapy: effect on disabilities of patients with total hip arthroplasty", Archives of Physical Medicine and Rehabilitation, vol. 77, no. 3, pp. 273-277.

Shih, C.H., Du, Y.K., Lin, Y.H. & Wu, C.C. 1994, "Muscular recovery around the hip joint after total hip arthroplasty", Clinical orthopaedics and related research, vol. (302), no. 302, pp. 115-120.

Sinaki, M. 2004, "Falls, fractures, and hip pads", Current osteoporosis reports, vol. 2, no. 4, pp. 131-137.

Skelton, D.A., Greig, C.A., Davies, J.M. & Young, A. 1994, "Strength, power and related functional ability of healthy people aged 65-89 years", Age and Ageing, vol. 23, no. 5, pp. 371-377.

Stratford, P.W., Kennedy, D., Pagura, S.M. & Gollish, J.D. 2003, "The relationship between self-report and performance-related measures: questioning the content validity of timed tests", Arthritis and Rheumatism, vol. 49, no. 4, pp. 535-540.

Suetta, C., Andersen, J.L., Dalgas, U., Berget, J., Koskinen, S., Aagaard, P., Magnusson, S.P. & Kjaer, M. 2008, "Resistance training induces qualitative changes in muscle morphology, muscle architecture, and muscle function in elderly postoperative patients", Journal of applied physiology (Bethesda, Md.: 1985), vol. 105, no. 1, pp. 180-186.

Suetta, C., Magnusson, S.P., Rosted, A., Aagaard, P., Jakobsen, A.K., Larsen, L.H., Duus, B. & Kjaer, M. 2004, "Resistance training in the early postoperative phase reduces hospitalization and leads to muscle hypertrophy in elderly hip surgery patients--a controlled, randomized study", Journal of the American Geriatrics Society, vol. 52, no. 12, pp. 2016-2022.

Terwee, C.B., Mokkink, L.B., Steultjens, M.P. & Dekker, J. 2006, "Performance-based methods for measuring the physical function of patients with osteoarthritis of the hip or knee: a systematic review of measurement properties", *Rheumatology (Oxford, England)*, vol. 45, no. 7, pp. 890-902.

Trudelle-Jackson, E., Emerson, R. & Smith, S. 2002, "Outcomes of total hip arthroplasty: a study of patients one year postsurgery", The Journal of orthopaedic and sports physical therapy, vol. 32, no. 6, pp. 260-267.

Trudelle-Jackson, E. & Smith, S.S. 2004, "Effects of a late-phase exercise program after total hip arthroplasty: a randomized controlled trial", Archives of Physical Medicine and Rehabilitation, vol. 85, no. 7, pp. 1056-1062.

van Baar, M.E., Assendelft, W.J., Dekker, J., Oostendorp, R.A. & Bijlsma, J.W. 1999, "Effectiveness of exercise therapy in patients with osteoarthritis of the hip or knee: a systematic review of randomized clinical trials", Arthritis and Rheumatism, vol. 42, no. 7, pp. 1361-1369.

Wang, A.W., Gilbey, H.J. & Ackland, T.R. 2002, "Perioperative exercise programs improve early return of ambulatory function after total hip arthroplasty: a randomized, controlled trial", American Journal of Physical Medicine & Rehabilitation / Association of Academic Physiatrists, vol. 81, no. 11, pp. 801-806.

Wang, B.W., Ramey, D.R., Schettler, J.D., Hubert, H.B. & Fries, J.F. 2002, "Postponed development of disability in elderly runners: a 13-year longitudinal study", Archives of Internal Medicine, vol. 162, no. 20, pp. 2285-2294.

Wang, W., Morrison, T.A., Geller, J.A., Yoon, R.S. & Macaulay, W. 2009, "Predicting Short-Term Outcome of Primary Total Hip Arthroplasty A Prospective Multivariate Regression Analysis of 12 Independent Factors", The Journal of arthroplasty, .

Ware, J.E.,Jr & Sherbourne, C.D. 1992, "The MOS 36-item short-form health survey (SF-36). I. Conceptual framework and item selection", *Medical care*, vol. 30, no. 6, pp. 473-483.

Ware, J.,Jr, Kosinski, M. & Keller, S.D. 1996, "A 12-Item Short-Form Health Survey: construction of scales and preliminary tests of reliability and validity", *Medical care*, vol. 34, no. 3, pp. 220-233.

Wigerstad-Lossing, I., Grimby, G., Jonsson, T., Morelli, B., Peterson, L. & Renstrom, P. 1988, "Effects of electrical muscle stimulation combined with voluntary contractions after knee ligament surgery", Medicine and science in sports and exercise, vol. 20, no. 1, pp. 93-98.

Wijgman, A.J., Dekkers, G.H., Waltje, E., Krekels, T. & Arens, H.J. 1994, "No positive effect of preoperative exercise therapy and teaching in patients to be subjected to hip arthroplasty", Nederlands tijdschrift voor geneeskunde, vol. 138, no. 19, pp. 949-952.

Wilson, J., Charlett, A., Leong, G., McDougall, C. & Duckworth, G. 2008, "Rates of surgical site infection after hip replacement as a hospital performance indicator: analysis of data from the English mandatory surveillance system", Infection control and hospital epidemiology : the official journal of the Society of Hospital Epidemiologists of America, vol. 29, no. 3, pp. 219-226.

Wood, G.C. & McLauchlan, G.J. 2006, "Outcome assessment in the elderly after total hip arthroplasty", The Journal of arthroplasty, vol. 21, no. 3, pp. 398-404.

Young, N.L., Cheah, D., Waddell, J.P. & Wright, J.G. 1998, "Patient characteristics that affect the outcome of total hip arthroplasty: a review", Canadian journal of surgery.Journal canadien de chirurgie, vol. 41, no. 3, pp. 188-195.

8

Rehabilitation of Patients Following Arthroplasty of the Hip and Knee

Magdalena Wilk-Frańczuk
Frycz-Modrzewski Cracow University,
Cracow Rehabilitation Center, Scanmed St. Rafael Hospital, Cracow
Poland

1. Introduction

Arthroplasty (Latin arthroplastica) with endoprosthesis is a reconstructive procedure whose purpose is to restore the damaged joint by creating a substitute joint with actions similar to those of the physiological joint. The term "arthroplasty" is used interchangeably in the literature with "total joint replacement" or "alloplasty."

There are several indications for arthroplasty, especially involving the large joints of the lower limbs, such as hip or knee, which are exposed to significant loads. Total joint replacement is mainly applied to joints damaged by a disease process (e.g. osteoarthritis). Arthroplasties are performed in people of all ages; however, elderly patients make up the majority. Primarily cemented or uncemented prostheses are implanted, rarely the so-called hybrid type, where only one element is embedded in bone cement. Regardless of the type of prosthesis, however, or its construction, the operated joint, or the surgical approaches used, as well as the patient's age, Body Mass Index (BMI), or general state of health, each patient needs an adequate rehabilitation protocol. This protocol should be instituted before surgery, or immediately after if the operation is performed on an emergency basis.

Since the application of the first prosthesis, there has been continuous progress in this field. This applies to the materials and design of the prostheses, the surgical techniques used, and post-operative rehabilitation. The largest differences relate to the point at which physiotherapy begins and (and perhaps most importantly) when the patient stands up and full weight is put on the joint. The physician, usually the orthopedic surgeon who performed the operation, makes the decision to implement rehabilitation. But the decision as to when to stand the patient up and the assessment of the load capacity of the operated limb also belong to physiotherapist.

Close interdisciplinary cooperation is always of great importance for the patient, in this case the patient after arthroplasty, who often requires an individual rehabilitation program (Grotle et al., 2010). This individualization involves some modifications of the general scheme of rehabilitation developed and used in orthopedic and rehabilitation centers. After standard operations, the early full loading of the operated limb gives much better post-operative results, and the patient regains functional capacity sooner. Outcome assessment should be monitored. Studies have used different research methods, including the functional evaluation of patients using different scales, such as the Harris scale, a 100-point scale that assesses the quality of life especially of older patients, as well as the impact of various factors such as BMI on the healing process (Cichy et al., 2008; Dudda et al., 2010; Starowicz et al., 2005). In addition to standard physiotherapy assessment instruments, methods based on computer analysis use dedicated equipment and computer programs (e.g. stabilometry platforms, sEMG, strain gauge tests, photoelastic tests, pedobarography, and thermal tests – Burnfield et al., 2010; Cichy & Wilk, 2006; Cichy et al., 2008; Maguire et al., 2010; Wilk et al., 2004, 2008). This allows for more objective results, and also leads to the formulation of new ideas for modifying and optimizing patient rehabilitation programs.

2. Rehabilitation after hip arthroplasty

Arthroplasty with prosthesis, or total hip replacement with an artificial joint to replace the one that has been destroyed, has ushered in a new era in the treatment of degenerative arthritis. The occurrence of osteoarthritis seems to be a consequence of the European style of civilization, as it almost does not occur in India, Mexico, South America, Africa, or the Far East (except for Japan and Australia). In Poland, according to epidemiological studies by various authors, osteoarthritis affects approximately 10 to 20% of the population, and therefore between 4 and 8 million people, including approximately 4% between 18 and 34 years of age and up to 85% of people over the age of 75. From the clinical point of view, and in terms of frequency, osteoarthritis of the hip occupies a prominent place next to osteoarthritis of the knee and spinal joints. It is characterized by localized pain in the groin area, on the front or side of the thigh, and is often associated with radiating pain around the knee. These symptoms appear and worsen after exercise, or a longer walk, but often also occur at rest and at night. There is stiffness in the morning or after prolonged immobilization of the joint, and the dysfunction is often associated with swelling, limited range of motion, muscle weakness, and radiographic changes.

The etiology of osteoarthritis of the hip is easy to determine if the patient has a congenital or acquired defect during development, such as hip dysplasia, Perthes disease, or deformity of the femoral head. Some other factors that are easy to determine are adverse biochemical changes occurring in articular cartilage, or a dislocation or fracture within the joint in the past. Frequently, however, the cause of the disease remains difficult to establish, because degenerative-deforming hip joint diseases are not an homogeneous disease entity, but a complex of lesions arising as a result of different causal factors. Given the diversity of these factors, degenerative-deforming changes of the hip joints can be divided into two basic groups: - primary (idiopathic) coxarthrosis and secondary coxarthrosis. The first group includes patients diagnosed on the basis of clinical examinations, along with radiological and laboratory tests. and cannot be said to prove the root cause of the disease. The second group are patients with, for example, congenital or acquired hip disorders.

The diagnostic criteria for primary hip osteoarthritis adopted and published in 2000 by the American College of Rheumatology include pain in the joint and at least two of the three following symptoms: ESR <20 mm after 1 hour; edge or central osteophytes detected radiographically; joint space stenosis (Moody, 2000).

The degenerative process is irreversible. However, appropriately individualized and systematic conservative treatment helps to reduce pain, maintain range of motion, and increase muscle strength, thereby reducing disability and slowing the progression of the disease. This treatment involves the use of NSAIDs and analgesics, and an appropriate rehabilitation program, which consists of physical treatments, kinesitherapy, and if necessary the selection of appropriate auxiliary orthopedic equipment (canes, crutches, walkers). Possible supplements include occupational therapy and education involving the patients and their families, to make them familiar with the specific nature of the disease, ongoing conservative treatment, prevention, and surgical options.

Unfortunately, conservative treatment of osteoarthritis only slows the progress of the disease, and is therefore associated with the slow deterioration of the patients' overall efficiency and their ability to perform activities of daily living, such as walking, washing, performing physiological functions without assistance, dressing, preparing meals, etc. That is why a person who has severe pain while walking, even when at rest, and significant motor deficits, even with small radiographic changes, requires surgical treatment. The method of choice is the replacement of the overused or damaged joint with an artificial one. In the overwhelming number of cases this concerns older patients (over 65 years of age), especially women (at a ratio of 3:1). Hip prosthesis implantation in these patients has now become standard procedure in Poland and worldwide.

The creator of replacement arthroplasty is considered historically to be Themistocles Gluck, who in 1891 developed and implanted the first artificial ball-and-socket joint. Further studies were focused on finding new materials for the implants, new models and surgical techniques. The most significant development of hip joint replacement began in the 1960s and continues until today. The founder of modern total joint replacement is J. Charnley, who made the first implantation of a hip prosthesis with a polyethylene acetabulum. Since 1951, polymethylmethacrylate has been used as bone cement for fixing cemented prostheses. However, a fundamental feature of this cement is its "aging," as evidenced by the occurrence of cracking and irritation due to reactive granulation tissue, which separates the cement from the bone, leading to loosening of the prosthesis. The development of technology and operating methods did not produce improved rehabilitation until the 1980s. In general, cemented prostheses are used to treat older patients, for whom early mobilization is important with full weight bearing during ambulation with both lower limbs. This is important because of age-related, physiological changes in motor coordination and muscle strength and to prevent complications from the respiratory and circulatory systems.

The first cementless prosthesis was applied in the 1980s. These prostheses are designed for young people with the potential for regeneration and osteogenesis of the bone, and good structural conditions of the acetabulum and femur. The construction of cementless endoprostheses is intended to match the material to the biological and strength features of the bone. The fastening elements of cementless prostheses are the result of many studies, which have recently led to the creation of threaded or press-fitted cups. The construction and method of mounting screwed-in and press-fitted prostheses produces good stabilization and the ability to distribute forces evenly over the entire length of the stem and acetabular surface, which also allows for quick loading of the limb.

The further development of arthroplasty depends primarily on interdisciplinary cooperation with physicians, engineers, and physiotherapists. The introduction of the implant to the bone always changes the distribution of internal stresses. Biomechanical studies (Będziński & Ścigała, 2000) on the effects of various types of endoprosthesis stems on the strain in the shaft of the femur showed non-physiological stress distribution and deformation of bone tissue in the case of long stems. Recently short-stemmed prostheses allow for a more favorable distribution of bone strain and smaller overloads in some areas within the femur when loading the lower limb. Evaluation of the results of surgical treatment and rehabilitation with the use of short-stem endoprosthesis shows a subjective reduction in pain intensity and less time to stand up and learn to walk, which is beneficial for speeding up the healing process and returning the patient to independent performance of activities of daily life after 4 - 8 weeks. This is also a financial issue (shorter hospital stay, no need for third party assistance, etc.).

Development of the stem design for the hip prosthesis has been moving in the direction of shorter and smaller stems, in which the stress distribution between implant-bone will allow the most accurate reproduction of physiological conditions. New solutions in hip surface replacement are also used for this purpose. In addition, the way of thinking has changed in favor of implanting a greater number of cementless prostheses in the elderly, whenever proper bone structure allows for such a possibility.

The criteria for evaluating treatment outcomes using endoprosthesis are the same for all stypes, and include the assessment of prosthesis stabilization, subjective sensations of pain, and functional capacity, as affected by muscle strength and range of motion. Muscle strength, an important factor for functional capabilities, depends partly on individual and hereditary characteristics, such as the cross section of the muscle and its structure, but primarily on the level of physical activity (Wilk et al., 2004; Wilk & Frańczuk, 2003, 2005a; Wilk-Frańczuk et al., 2011). The latter develops and takes shape during normal human development. Rapid increases in muscle strength begin in boys at age 13-14 and lasts until age 19-20. In later years (after age 30) it remains constant, then decreases. In girls, the stabilization of muscle strength occurs after puberty. As a result of the processes of human aging, physical capacity gradually decreases. Between the ages of 20 and 30 years, skeletal muscles make up about 45% of the human body, but after 70 years of age, only 27%. The decrease in muscle strength (about 1% per year) as a result of the process of aging is caused primarily by progressive muscle atrophy and changes occurring in peripheral nerves. This leads to limitations, and even loss of locomotion, which is a serious problem because it leads to a decrease in the cardio-pulmonary exercise capacity of the patient and the development of metabolic diseases. In the United States, research on the effects of rehabilitation combined with strength training for older people found that even at the age of 90 it is possible to increase isometric force, slow down significantly the loss of muscle mass, and enhance locomotor capabilities.

In the case of hip arthroplasty with a prosthesis, functional outcome seems to be the most convincing parameter of assessment, hence early and appropriate rehabilitation is very important to obtain the best functional outcome, as we have emphasized above. Arthroplasty, by eliminating pain and increasing the range of motion in the joint that is reduced by osteoarthritis, allows training to be intensified, which increases muscle mass and strength. Thus the patient gets, in addition to pain relief, the possibility of recovering locomotion, and thereby obtains greater functional efficiency and an important factor contributing to a higher quality of life (QOL). Patient assessment from this point of view is rare in the literature, where most of the authors work on a variety of point-scales, taking into account the local and overall efficiency of the patient, and in some cases also the radiological picture. For many years the basic, relatively simple method of evaluating the functional status of the patient after surgery arthroplasty was the Charnley or Harris test. This assessment is still widely used as an additional outcome measure. The value of the Harris scale (Harris Hip Score) has been well documented in the literature (the scale has been in use since 1969). It also features very reproducible results, and the evaluation includes the assessment ofQOL parameters. The Harris scale assesses the following groups of parameters: pain (intensity, medications used); gait (limping, use of crutches or canes, walking distance); performance of daily activities (climbing stairs, sitting, tying shoes); ability to use public transport; hip range of motion (detailed ranges); presence or absence of deformities (contractures or shortening of the limb).

The end result of the evaluation of individual parameters is a sub-point value, all of which when added give the total score on a scale from 0 to 100 points.

A number of other scales have been developed for the clinical evaluation of patients with osteoarthritis of the hip, before and after surgery. Currently in use, in addition to the aforementioned Harris scale, are the Merle d'Aubigne-Postel scale, the Bellamy scale, the WOMAC scale (Western Ontario and McMasters Universities Questionnaire), whose particular advantage is allowing the patient to make a self-assessment, the JOA scale (Japanese Orthopaedic Association), the Wolfe scale, and the Lequesne scale.

Technological progress has made it possible to develop more objective methods for assessing the results of arthroplasty. These include the assessment of gait parameters. The basic parameters initially used to evaluate gait basic included gait speed, step frequency, and step length, measured by means of micro switches attached to the patient's shoes. In subsequent years there has been a new method to identify and assess the symmetry of the lower limbs and gait cycle phases using miniature accelerometers. There is also a more thorough analysis of gait using a series of images made with the patient walking, at a frequency from 300 to 1200 shots per minute, or even something as unusual as the method developed by Bergman's team, based on the implantation of a prosthesis fitted with a telemetry transmitter. Another contemporary method is to measure ground reaction forces during gait using dynamographic platforms. These allow us to measure ground reaction forces in all directions and linear momentum, and therefore to assess the accuracy of limb loading when walking. Currently, the latest optical electronic devices have been used to develop gait analysis systems for registering the movement trajectory of markers placed on the patient, often with the addition of integrated graphics platforms, known as dynamographic platforms. There are also other devices, such as, for example, gas meters for measuring oxygen and carbon dioxide in exhaled air, and electromyography.

Such tests allow us to collect a large amount of information; however, they are feasible only in specialized laboratories and report only the overall efficiency of the system. Assessment by these means is incomplete and does not affect measurements of range of motion in the operated joint and the pelvic girdle muscle forces responsible for individual movements. Such studies may be more useful for assessing the efficiency of locomotion, and indirectly serve to evaluate the use of implants, but they do not return function and muscle strength. Recently, encouraging results of functional assessment of muscles and ranges of motion after implantation of prostheses in the operated limb have been obtained using the technique of wireless surface electromyography – sEMG (Maguire et al., 2010).

There is no generally accepted rehabilitation protocol for patients after total hip replacement with cemented or cementless prosthesis. The differences relate to both the methods of rehabilitation and the date of commencement of full loading of the operated joint (Iyengar et al., 2007; Wilk & Frańczuk, 2005a). A constant search for optimal solutions is therefore necessary. Rehabilitation after cemented hip arthroplasty starts from the first day after surgery with the introduction of breathing exercises. The second day begins with isometric exercises, passive-active exercises of the operated limb, active exercises of the unaffected limb and upper limbs. On the third day we begin to stand the patients up and teach them to walk with crutches or a walker with no weight bearing. What is most preferred, however, is for the patient to behave consistently with the features of normal gait - the operated foot is put on the ground with no weight bearing. At the end of the first week after the operation, gradual loading of the operated limb begins, starting with 20-30% of body weight. A weight training floor is most often used to teach the patient the proper balance of body weight. Full weight bearing is applied after the stitches have been removed.

In the case of cementless hip arthroplasty, all motor activity is often delayed. Exercises usually begin on the first day, but the patient stands for the first time on the 5th to 14th day after surgery, and partial loading of the operated limb starts 4-6 weeks after surgery, with full weight bearing after 3-4 months. Some authors recommend no weight bearing for up to 6 months, although others support full weight bearing as soon as possible (2-3 days after surgery), especially when screwed-in implants have been used (e.g. Zweymüller-Stemcup). In general, in the first weeks after arthroplasty the appropriate positioning of the operated limb is recommended - slight adduction, 5 degree hip and knee flexion, neutral rotation position. Excessive abduction, internal rotation and crossing the legs are contraindicated.

Based on many years of research and observation, I believe that after the standard procedure, when the prosthesis is properly implanted, the rehabilitation protocol for both cemented and cementless prostheses should be the same, and include early loading of the operated limb (Cichy et al., 2008; Wilk & Frańczuk, 2003, 2004). This does not apply to non-standard patients (extra implants strengthening the acetabulum, bone grafts, proximal femur fracture fixation, etc.). Limb loading in these cases is delayed; the patients usually walk with crutches till the bone is healed, and after that gradual weight bearing is introduced. It is best to start learning before surgery.

It has been shown that in the first period after surgery the greatest impact on the progress of rehabilitation results from: minimally invasive surgery within the interval between the tensor fasciae latae, rectus femoris and sartorius muscles, or within the interval between the tensor fasciae latae and gluteus medius muscles; epidural analgesia in the first 24 hours after surgery; the use of Continuous Passive Motion (CPM) in the first days after surgery.

In contrast to arthroplasty performed with minimally invasive approaches, the other operating approaches require a delay in the entire rehabilitation process, mainly related to standing the patient up and teaching ambulation, even by a few weeks, because premature active rehabilitation in the first weeks after surgery can lead to dislocation of the implant (Dudda et al., 2008). The type of implanted prosthesis may also affect postoperative functionality.

A common problem after total hip replacement is a subjective sense of unequal length of the legs. If there is no actual reduction in the relative limb length, one should take into account the possibility of pelvic positioning dysfunction, which can be expressed by the asymmetry of iliac spine positioning (anterior superior and posterior superior). Asymmetrical muscle tone can be the cause of this.

About 1100 hip and knee replacements per year are done in our center (the Cracow Rehabilitation Center). Lateral or antero-lateral approaches are routinely used for hip replacement, and the anterior approach with ischemia for knee replacement. The mean operating time for this type of treatment varies between 45 and 60 minutes, with spinal anesthesia, and the patients are subjected to a constant process of rehabilitation. Before the operation the patients are informed about the stages of rehabilitation that will follow, and learn to walk on crutches with different loads on the lower limbs, which increases their conscious and active participation in the treatment process.

On the first post-operative day CPM is introduced, which improves the limb blood supply, accelerates the absorption of the hematoma, reduces the hypertonicity of periarticular tissues, and allows the patient to get rid of the anxiety associated with the movement of the operated joint. In subsequent days, exercises are gradually introduced, applying the principles of individualization and gradation of difficulty. On the third day, walking re-education begins, with gradually increasing weight bearing and the use of appropriate orthopedic aids (walker, crutches). Due to the fact that arthroplasty is most often related to a chronic degenerative process, which also causes major progressive pathological changes in connective tissue and contributes to a significant reduction in patient activity, special attention is paid to the restoration of normal movement patterns. It is also essential to learn to maintain and control proper posture, which may be disturbed due to the abnormal movement patterns both before and after surgery (e.g. due to the constant need to relieve one leg, abnormal movement with the use of one crutch).

One of the characteristic features of degenerative joint diseases is that only a relatively small percentage of the patients who present for treatment (8-10%) are vocationally active. Many studies have shown that once patients have been relieved of their pain symptoms, they are more willing to exercise and become physically active. It is also important to draw attention to the analysis of treatment outcomes in the first period after surgery. This period is especially important, since exercises can be intensified immediately after surgery, and it is during this period that CPM can be applied most effectively. In any event, the impact of the latter is not perceptible at a later stage. Early rehabilitation (especially CPM), commenced immediately after surgery, along with appropriate pharmacotherapy and the application of elastic pressure stockings on the lower limbs, also helps to prevent such complications as pneumonia, venous embolisms or thrombosis. This is consistent with the observations of other authors. The results of studies on muscle strength suggest that muscle strength begins to recover about 3 months after surgery, while an appropriate program of rehabilitation can lead to increased muscle strength within 6 months. This observation is confirmed by the analysis of range of motion. When functionality is evaluated according to the Merle D'Aubigne functional scale, published research results indicate that a distinct majority of patients recover good functionality in the operated limb after six months. These results are similar to those obtained in respect to muscle strength, although they do not in fact show the dynamics of change in respect to either muscle strength or range of motion.

In the prevention of disorders of posture, those patients who will have to use elbow crutches for a longer period of time are advised to use two crutches rather than one, which affects the symmetry of body work during ambulation. Approximately one week after surgery, the patient learns to walk up and down stairs, initially leading with the non-operated limb while going up, and with the operated limb while going down. Throughout the period of treatment we adapt the rehabilitation program to the individual patient, and where indicated we use other physiotherapeutic methods (e.g. physical agents).

The rehabilitation applied initially in the orthopedic department should be continued later at home, with the cooperation of the family, or, if that is not possible, in a medical rehabilitation unit (Iyengar et al., 2007). The lack of appropriate rehabilitation in this early period can often seriously undermine the effects of the surgeon's efforts. In the later, post-discharge period, our patients are often advised to try Nordic Walking.

3. Rehabilitation after arthroplasty of the knee

From the clinical point of view, as previously stated, gonarthrosis, along with coxarthrosis and spondylarthrosis, is among the most significant joint pathologies. When the changes are significant, gonarthrosis can be handicapping, while pain occurs with even minor deviations from the physiological norm. In most cases the causes of the disease are difficult to determine, since degenerative and deformative changes do not constitute a unified nosological entity, but rather a syndrome of pathological changes caused by the operation of various etiological factors. Research has shown that gonarthrosis does not affect only the elderly, since degenerative changes in the knee also occur in much younger persons. Among the generally recognized risk factors are the following: abnormalities in joint structure; biomechanical disturbances; overloading of the joint; microlesions; obesity.

Gonarthrosis can also be caused by deformities (varus more often than valgus), which cause one of the joint components to be overloaded. Conservative treatment consists in rehabilitation and pharmacotherapy, while patients are advised to adopt a conservative lifestyle and lose weight. The degenerative process that has begun is slowed down under the influence of conservative treatment, but even so the changes tend to progress. As in the case of hip arthroplasty, the appearance of severe pain that occurs both during ambulation and at rest, along with restricted range of motion in the knees, eventually leads to a significant degree of disability. In that situation, the treatment of choice is surgery, involving the replacement of the damaged joint with an artificial one.

The physiological exhaustion of tissue that is characteristic of aging, especially in the weight-bearing joints, is one of the most commonly cited causes of primary degenerative disease of the largest joint in the human body, the knee. The external loads on this joint that result from the forces of gravity and ground reaction are to a large extent dependent on body mass. The load on the joint in standing position constitutes approximately 43% of body weight (Kabsch & Bober, 2001). During ambulation, the pressure on the joint surfaces changes depending on the gait phase: the greatest load occurs at the beginning of the support phase. These parameters can also change in the event of varus or valgus deformations of the joint, which amplify the pressure on the most heavily loaded parts of the joint. Biomechanical research has produced different models of knee joint loading (the Maquet model, the Denham model), taking account of assymetrical loads on joint surfaces in the case of varus or valgus deformities of the lower joints. Indeed, such deformities are among the indications for surgical treatment. When the angle of deviation is not too great, correctional popliteal osteotomy of the tibia is applied. Deformities that produce a greater angle of deviation require arthroplasty with endoprosthesis, especially when they are accompanied by deformities of the joint surfaces.

As in the case of the hip joint, the increased number of knee arthroplasties performed in the last decade has produced a search for new solutions in surgery and rehabilitation. The first knee endoprostheses were implanted in the 1950s, when a leading role in their development was played by Smith-Petersen, Waldius, and Campbell, among others. These prostheses had a hinge construction, which often caused early loosening. In the 1960s and 70s, new types of prosthesis were introduced. In 1971, the Canadian surgeon Frank H. Gunston, who was cooperating at that time with Sir John Charnley on a new type of hip prosthesis (consisting of a metal femoral part mounted on bone cement and a polyethylene acetabulum), developed a polycentric knee prosthesis, based on their joint research. Since that time there has been constant progress, thanks to research on improving the construction of the prosthesis in such a way as to reproduce most accurately the movement of a natural joint, and on the application of construction materials that are as biocompatibile as possible. Many prosthesis models have been designed, two of which are currently most often used: mobile-bearing and fixed-bearing, posterior stabilized with a pin to replace the functions of the posterior cruciate ligament. Among these designs there are many types of prostheses that can be adapted to the individual patient, including, for example, unicompartmental prostheses (Zeni & Snyder-Mackler, 2010).

Both types of prosthesis, mobile-bearing and fixed-bearing, have their adherents. In the case of mobile-bearing prostheses, what is emphasized is the possibility to achieve a greater range of flexion in the knee joint and a physiological gait. Fixed-bearing prostheses, in turn, provide greater possibilities to correct deformities in the knee joint, but they can also cause shearing forces to develop, which can lead to loosening of the joint. However, it is often emphasized in the literature that the frequency of occurrence of loosening in both types of prosthesis is comparable. On the other hand, in the case of the knee joint, the implantation of a prothesis with a modeling system that uses an MRI of the lower limb reduces bleeding (since it is then unnecessary to open the medullary canal), shortens operating time, and, as indicated by preliminary studies, makes it possible to obtain better outcomes, in terms of a quicker recovery of full functionality of the operated limb.

Progress and the development of knee arthroplasty with endoprosthesis has made it necessary to adapt rehabilitation procedures, so as to obtain the best possible outcome for the patient. There are many different factors, before, during, and after surgery, that can affect the treatment outcome; the primary goal of the surgery itself is to reduce pain and increase the range of motion in the limb affected by pathological changes. These two effects, in turn, are intended to promote recovery of normal gait, thereby allowing the patient to regain functional independence and normal activity in daily life, which is a major factor in QOL. It should be obvious, then, that proper rehabilitation, adapted to the individual needs and capabilities of the patient and to contemporary standards of practice, plays a very significant role in outcome. In publications from as late as the mid-1990s, there are still descriptions of post-operative rehabilitation that began on the 2nd or 3rd day after surgery with kinesitherapy (active-passive and passive exercises), becoming gradually more intensive over the next several days. It was only on the 8th day after surgery that the patient was encouraged to sit on the edge of the bed, and on the 10th day that the first attempt was made to stand the patient up, followed by ambulation training from the 12th to the 14th day (Nolewajek et al., 2008), who studied the risk factors for deep vein thrombosis in the lower limbs in patients after total knee arthroplasty, found that the time when the patient first stands up is of major importance in the prevention of embolic or thrombotic complications, alongside age, obesity, and duration of surgery. Rehabilitation after arthroplasty of the knee is oriented primarily towards allowing the patient to return to normal activities of daily living and functional independence as soon as possible.

An appropriate program of rehabilitation is thus an essential element in treatment, to prepare the patient for surgery and after surgery, with the goal of standing the patient up as soon as possible, teaching ambulation, and recovering as much functionality as possible. The rehabilitation process is often lengthy, and the patient's physical fitness before surgery is of no small importance. Currently, given the necessity to adapt the rehabilitation program to each individual patient, rehabilitation begins on the 1st or 2nd day post-operatively, with respiratory exercises and isometrics, accompanied by active-passive and active exercises.

The patient stands for the first time on the 2nd or 3rd day post-operatively, initially with a high walking platform, followed by ambulation training with elbow crutches. On the 7th to 9th day post-operatively the patient begins to learn how to walk up and down stairs, and then, depending on the patient's fitness and gait mechanics with crutches, two-beat ambulation with a single elbow crutch on the arm contralateral to the operated knee. It is essential, however, to pay attention to the patient's body posture in motion, and if asymmetrical shoulder positioning is observed during ambulation with one crutch, then the use of two crutches is recommended. Just as in the case of hip replacement surgery, this prevents the patient from becoming accustomed to an abnormal pattern of motion.

The rehabilitation of patients after total knee arthroplasty is a complex task for the physiotherapist. An important goal is to achieve full extension of the joint and the greatest possible flexion. This task is rendered all the more difficult by the fact that practically every patient has pain symptoms that hinder or prevent intensive kinesitherapy. Pain reduction, then, can be regarded as the first goal of rehabilitation. An analysis of the impact of low temperatures on the human body leads to the conclusion that its analgesic effect is the one felt most quickly. In the research group, this effect was noted in all patients. The analgesic effect has been observed by many authors, in respect to different joints (knee, hip). The research performed first by our group on the application of local cryotherapy in the treatment of painful shoulder syndrome has shown that this method makes a major contribution to eliminating pain, which makes it possible to implement therapeutic exercises at an early stage. Under the influence of pain, a vicious circle often forms: pain causes a limited range of mobility in the joint, which leads to increased muscle tension and further limitation of motion, steadily increasing the level of pain.

The implementation of a systematic rehabilitation program for patients after total knee arthroplasty, both cemented and cementless, not only produces good outcomes, but also, as in the case of other surgical procedures, prevents complications. Among the rehabilitation techniques used with knee arthroplasty patients there are some special methods, such as CPM, biological feedback devices, or physicotherapy, especially local cryotherapy (Wilk & Frańczuk, 2004, 2005a, 2005b). Disturbances of proprioception after surgery render it necessary to include exercises in a closed kinematic chain and exercises to correct equilibrium in the later stage of the rehabilitation program.

Stabilometric platforms or parapodiums are very useful for evaluating equilibrium in patients recovering from total knee arthroplasty. These devices, in addition to teaching various activities, often connected with biofeedback, can also provide an objective evaluation of treatment outcome. The application of rotors with computer analysis of training supports the proper training of the symmetrical work of the lower limbs after total knee arthroplasty.

4. Rehabilitation after arthroplasty of the hip or knee in older patients

The increasing percentage of older persons in the general population is making it essential to search diligently for ways to preserve a level of fitness that would allow functional independence to be preserved, even in advanced old age (Marks, 2010). At present the maximum duration of human life is estimated at 110-120 years (though there are persons who live longer, and there are frequent news reports about persons who are older yet), but this pertains to persons characterized by exceptional genetic traits, and is also conditioned by biological and environmental conditions. An example of this problem might be the more than 100,000 centenarians living in Japan, as compared to some African countries, where the average life expectancy does not exceed 50 years. Still, given the increasing life expectancy, the literature increasingly divides the older population into three separate age brackets: the "young-old" (65-74), the "old old" (75-84), and the "oldest old" (over 85) (Evgeniadis et al., 2008; Wilk-Frańczuk et al., 2011; Wright et al., 2011). This increasing life span, undoubtedly related to the progress of civilization, including advances in medicine, means that more and more people are reaching the age of 65 in much better health than was the case in previous generations. Women continue to make up a majority of the older population, since their life expectancy is several years longer on the average than that of men. However, research performed with a group of 94 centenarians showed that the men in this group, though they made up only 12% of the whole group, were in better physical condition and generally led a more active life.

In spite of the fact that a constantly growing number of older persons are fitter and more active than before, still, the progress of involutionary processes in physiological aging causes limitations and poses numerous problems, especially after age 75. The frequent co-occurrence of several pathological processes with the physiological changes of normal aging often makes diagnosis and treatment difficult. The problems are compounded by deteriorating sensory perception and frequent depressive episodes, which renders it necessary to make medical personnel aware of the differences in the course of disease and associated treatment in the elderly patient.

One of the basic goals of treatment is to make it possible for the older person to return to independence in activities of daily living. This is conditional upon good health, and fundamentally affects the quality of life. The period during which the patient is dependent upon someone else should be as short as possible, and the family's support should be oriented towards motivating the patient to return to health. The primary means to achieving the greatest possible functionality and maintaining it throughout the lifespan is comprehensive rehabilitation, understood both as the sum of all its components, and as a model of procedure. The individualization of this process is particularly essential in older patients, especially in respect to the possibility of conducting parts of the rehabilitation program in the patient's home or in the form of ambulatory rehabilitation. This reduces the appearance of cognitive and emotional disturbances associated with the stress that is caused by being away from home, in an unfamiliar place. Older patients are often reluctant to agree to hospitalization, since for them the hospital is associated with serious illness and death. In situations where a hospital stay is inevitable, for example when surgery is necessary, its duration should be as brief as possible.

Currently, modern rehabilitation is creating conditions for standing the patients up and teaching them to walk as early as possible. In older persons with deformative and degenerative changes, eliminating pain and increasing locomotor capacity, in terms of gait ergonomics and efficiency, is of crucial importance to quality of life. One of the factors that has the most influence on the whole course of rehabilitation is the possibility of full weight bearing on the operated limb at the earliest possible moment. Another factor that reduces the number of potential fatal post-operative complications has been the introduction, since the beginning of this century, of preventive measures against thrombotic and embolic complications, not only in the form of low molecular weight heparin, but also thanks to changes in the philosophy of rehabilitation and a more active approach to elderly patients. This pertains not only to patients in orthopedic and traumatological wards, but also others, for example, patients in cardiological units after a heart attack. A more active and earlier rehabilitation based on early standing and the application of modern physiotherapeutic methods, such as CPM and other forms of kinesitherapy, has become something like a natural supplement to surgery. Of particular significance in this group of patients are the following: comprehensive, interdisciplinary preparation for surgery; rehabilitation that begins even before the operation; weight-bearing on the operated limb as soon as possible after surgery (Wilk & Frańczuk, 2004).

All of these factors contribute significantly to enabling the older patient to recover functionality, reducing the period of dependence on others, and improving the quality of life. The individualization of treatment, in turn, involves taking into account all dysfunctions and the level of mental and physical fitness, as well as the patient's involvement in planning rehabilitation. Currently, due to changes in both orthopedic procedures and rehabilitation, the mortality rate in this patient group is not high (several percent), and is more dependent on concomitant disorders in elderly patients, such as diabetes and other diseases, or dementia, which can hinder cooperation with medical personnel, or the medical history, than on the arthroplasty itself. This is also indicated by the results in hip arthroplasty that are now being achieved even in patients over 85 , the "oldest old". The final outcome of rehabilitation in these patients has not been observed to be significantly different from those of patients in other age brackets.

The rehabilitation program is always adapted to the current condition and subjective well-being of the patients, as well as their individual physical capacities. Before arthroplasty there are active, assisted, isometric, and respiratory exercises, along with positions and exercises to prevent edema. The patients are informed about what will happen after surgery, how soon they will stand and learn to walk, and about increasing weight-bearing on the operated lower limb with a walker and elbow crutches. All patients receive pharmacotherapy to prevent thrombosis for 14 days after surgery, while still hospitalized, using low molecular weight heparin administered subcutaneously (which is also continued after discharge, for an average of about 6 weeks). Elastic stockings are used in the perioperative period, and epidural anesthetics are also administered for a period of 48 hours after surgery. Rehabilitation commences on the first day after surgery, using respiratory exercises, which are continued as long as the patient remains on the ward. Next, on the second and third days, there are isometric and active-passive exercises for the operated limb, as well as CPM using electrical rail devices, such as the Artromot, Physiotek, or Canwell machines (extension and flexion of the hip with simultaneous flexion of the knee, and with the last-mentioned device, the ankle joint as well). The range of flexion in the hip joint is gradually increased to the extent possible given the patient's capacity. During this same period the patient gradually begins to stand, beginning with sitting on the edge of the bed, then standing beside the bed with a walker and learning to walk. As muscle function is recovered in the lower limb, the program is expanded to include assisted and active exercises, the walking distance is increased, and more weight is placed on the operated limb. On the 11th or 12th day after surgery, the first attempts are made to walk up and down stairs. There are two rehabilitation sessions daily (with CPM for 120-180 minutes a day), and after discharge the patient is instructed as to how to proceed further.

An important new direction for research in this area is the evaluation of posture stability, equilibrium, and displacing the center of gravity. For this purpose it is possible to use both clinical tests and appropriate devices, which often allow for a graphic display of the results. One example of this type of apparatus is the static-dynamic parapodium, to which a special computer program can be added, both to make a graphic representation of the results of rehabilitation and to provide exercises for the patient. Such devices can also be used to evaluate the risk of falls in those cases where the risk is greatest, i.e. with elderly patients. Thus the results of these tests can also have an indirect effect on the prevention of fractures (Wilk & Frańczuk, 2003; Wilk-Frańczuk et al., 2010).

As previously mentioned, the dysfunctional changes that occur with older patients co-occur with the physiological processes of aging. We are often dealing with the simultaneous appearance of different diseases associated with this period of life and those that occur in other age groups as well, which in the elderly may or may not show characteristic features. This co-occurrence of pathological changes often leads to handicap, which is especially true of disorders of the musculo-skeletal system, such as degenerative changes, rheumatoid arthritis, or osteoporotic fractures, as well as disorders of perception (Piva et al., 2011). That is why rehabilitation begins before the planned surgery, which makes it possible to prepare the patient and minimize anxiety about life after the surgery, through conscious planning of activities and the repetition of previously learned and already familiar patterns of motion. The changes occurring in old age, along with pathological changes that impair perception and the posture control system, lead to disregulation of stability, and often, as a result, to falls, which are the major internal cause of injuries and fractures in older persons (the external causes include environmental and situational factors). In as many as half of these patients, repeat injuries occur.

This problem also affects persons who have undergone arthroplasty, for whom the consequences of an injury are particularly dangerous due to their impact on the implant. Various parameters are used in tests involving the evaluation of equilibrium and stability in older persons, including especially the Tinetti test, the Duncan test, the Berg scale, or the Romberg maneuver. Nevertheless, for purposes of prevention in elderly patients it is essential to use methods and exercises aimed at improving equilibrium. The rehabilitation program should also include exercises to increase muscle strength in the upper limbs, especially the shoulders. This is very important for the patient's locomotion during the early post-operative period, when the patient is forced to move about on crutches. As in other age groups, walking on crutches should be symmetrical, preferably two-beat with symmetrical work of the upper limbs. Family support is also particularly important, oriented towards motivating the patient to take an active role in the process of treatment and supporting the patient's desire to recover fitness and health, and to continue rehabilitation later, at home (Iyengar et al., 2007).

5. Reeducation and methods of evaluating and testing gait

Walking is the most important means of human locomotion, and the inability to walk has a significant negative impact on QOL (Starowicz et al., 2005). Walking can be defined as a rhythmic, alternating movement of the lower limbs, combined with displacement of the trunk and concomitant movements of the upper limbs. During normal gait one lower limb is always in contact with the ground through the foot; what differentiates walking from running, then, is that in the former there is a phase of double support, which in running is replaced by a phase of flight.

Walking requires the simultaneous participation of all the joints in the lower limb in an extraordinarily complex movement chain. In addition, movements in the spinal joints, including the cervical segment, are of great importance, as are the alternating movements of the upper limbs. The involvement of all parts of the body in the mechanism of walking requires a well-coordinated, complicated control mechanism in the nervous system, which explains why walking is not possible immediately after birth, when the nervous system is not yet fully developed. Normal, physiological walking as a means of locomotion is extraordinarily energy efficient, which is why even slight disturbances increase the energy cost and reduce effectiveness. There are two phases in walking on a level surface when the energy cost is high. The first of these is when walking begins, when it is necessary to overcome inertia in order to displace body mass forward, and the second is stopping, when it is necessary to inhibit the movement of the limbs and trunk.

The kinematic pattern of normal gait is very similar in everyone. This is especially true of the movements that take place in all the joints involved in walking in the sagittal plane (e.g. in some people we can see greater deviations of the center of gravity while walking). The forces at work while walking result from the actions of muscles that evoke acceleration and slowing of the appropriate parts of the body, along with gravity and momentum. Walking is often described as an alternating process of losing and regaining equilibrium. Taking a step is associated with throwing the foot forward and displacing the body's center of gravity forward, which produces a loss of equilibrium. The forces of gravity and forward momentum cause a resultant continuation of the movement that has just begun. The fall is avoided by the reflex strategy of regaining equilibrium, i.e. the reaction of putting the foot on the floor, which is associated with the return of the center of gravity into the projection area of the rectangle of support. If walking is to be continued, the center of gravity must once again be displaced forward. During the next step, propulsion results from a much weaker contraction of the flexors in the calf of the leg, thanks to the momentum gained in the preceding step; then the body moves forward, and the next reflex step occurs. This mechanism is continued for as long as desired, and the momentum achieved allows for energy conservation as soon as an even cadence of successive steps is achieved.

The movement pattern in the hip joint is much less complex during walking than in the knee or ankle joints. In the entire walk cycle, the hip joint has one extension phase and one flexion stage, whereas the knee and ankle joints each perform two phases of each type in one cycle. However, while in the knee and ankle joints the range of motion involves only the sagittal plane (flexion and extension), the proper participation of the hip joint in walking requires a free range of motion in all three planes, since abduction, adduction, and rotation are elements of gait markers, i.e. factors contributing to the reduction of displacing the center of gravity. The limitation of abduction, adduction, and rotation results in the disruption of this mechanism, which is why the range of flexion and extension in the hip joint can often be preserved even when walking is impaired. When the heel strikes the ground, the hip joint is in light flexion, while the gluteus maximus and the posterior thigh muscles immediately contract, in order to initiate extension of the hip joint. The knee joint is in full extension or about 5° of flexion, while the posterior group of thigh muscles control the flexion of the knee that follows after the heel hits the ground. The upper ankle joint is in almost full dorsal flexion. When the body mass is shifted onto that limb, the group of hip adductors begins to act, followed almost immediately by the hip abductors, stabilizing the pelvis relative to the thigh. At the same time, the gluteus maximus tenses, extending the hip and stopping the internal rotation of the thigh. During the support phase, extension begins in the hip joint, as a result of the action of the extensor muscles; the knee joint increases its flexion in order to minimize the impact of the heel striking the ground and the vertical displacement of the center of gravity, which occurs when the weight of the body is displaced forward above the limb stabilized on the ground.

The flexion of the knee in the support phase is one of the classic gait markers, and can assume a value up to 30°. In the ankle joint, there is a controlled plantar flexion for safe release of the foot onto the ground. The contraction of the quadriceps softens the impact of the heel on the ground and controls the momentum of the body, now pushing the knee forward. In the support phase, the activity of the muscles virtually stops, with the exception of the calf muscles. This group begins to act during this phase, achieving its greatest activity just before the heel is lifted from the ground. The phase of taking the heel off the ground follows, as a result of propulsion and displacement of the center of gravity to the anterior part of the foot after full dorsal flexion of the foot has been obtained. Towards the end of this phase the contraction of the flexors of the foot adds the movement component necessary to push off from the ground. Then the hip adductors begin again, and the cycle starts all over.

The rehabilitation of arthroplasty patients should always be connected with reeducation in walking, preceded by a thorough evaluation of its mechanisms and existing disturbances of motion in the joints, and the activity of the particular muscles. The high degree of complication of the act of walking requires that it be divided into components for the sake of analysis. Some of the terminology pertains to the duration of particular phenomena, some to the spatial positions, the values of forces, and the distances covered by particular parts of the body (e.g. length of stride, length of the walk cycle, the walk cycle, its phases, speed, cadence, and gait markers). Gait disturbances can be viewed in both temporal and spatial relations, which is why a complete analysis must include both of these aspects. A complete gait analysis consists of the following: testing the force of pressure on the ground; a three-dimensional video record of the movement of the patient's anthropometric points; electromyographic tests of the activity of the muscles that participate in walking (Cichy & Wilk, 2006; Cichy et al., 2008; Giaquinto et al., 2007).

The application of all three of these elements gives the most complete picture of gait disturbances. Degenerative disease of both the hip joint and the knee joint significantly impairs the efficiency of gait, leading to a progressive deterioration of the quality of life.

Several specific groups of gait disorders can be noted in patients with osteoarthritis. These result from the major symptoms of osteoarthritis. The most striking change is slow gait, involving the ineffective use of momentum and greater fluctuations in the center of gravity in the sagittal plane. Pain in one of the lower limbs and reduced range of motion in the hip joint, in turn, result in gait impairment in the isometric aspect. So-called unisometric gait is present, and is characterized by impaired coordination, reduced duration of the support phase, shortening of stride length, shortening of the length of the affected limb and longer duration of the gait cycle. The most severe variant occurs when one of the lower limbs (mostly the affected one) is dragged forward, and only the healthy one is pushed forward. In pathological gait associated with osteoarthritis, deterioration of the isochronous aspect is also observed, which leads to to the formation of the so-called antalgic gait. The patient then prolongs the healthy limb support phase, in order to prepare the affected limb for contact with the ground, then "jumps" over the diseased limb and tries to put the healthy limb back on the ground. The impaired coordination of upper limb movements is associated with impaired balance and an asymmetrical loading pattern in both lower limbs.

The gait disturbances described above usually present simultaneously. Asymmetry of gait in patients with osteoarthritis of the hip has been noted (Cichy & Wilk, 2006). The asymmetry of the load on the lower limbs in a static test (while standing) is not detectable in patients, if shortening of the affected limb is not above 2 centimeters. When stride length is observed, changes have been detected in patients with osteoarthritis of the hip compared to a similar age group of the healthy population.

Gait re-education follows the principle of gradation of difficulty, and the program should also include improvement of balance and stability, so it is important to ensure patient safety (prevention of falls). Various methods are used to work with the patient, such as PNF, sensorimotor training, and hydrokinesitherapy. The rehabilitation program usually begins with exercises designed to achieve the correct loading of the lower limbs and gait pattern. Gradation is usually obtained by increasing the time of exercises, the number of repetitions, the distance, or by changing environmental conditions, such as walking on uneven ground, or walking outside the building. It is also important to introduce to the therapy elements of ordinary life, such as moving objects, and so called double tasks, which are intended to distract the patient who is focused on walking (simultaneous conversation, counting, observation, etc.).

6. Some special methods used in rehabilitation after total joint replacement

6.1 Continuous passive motion

Continuous Passive Motion (CPM) is one of many methods of rehabilitation after total joint replacement, which is the modern continuation of the G.J. Zander method, formerly known as mechanotherapy or the Zander method. One of the proponents and supporters of mechanotherapy is R.B. Salter, professor of orthopedic surgery in Toronto, who developed a method of continuous passive motion based on mechanical devices. From 1970 to 1986, Salter conducted research on the negative influence of immobilization on the joints, proving the beneficial effect of intermittent motion, and then continuous motion. In 1978 he constructed the first mechanical CPM device for patients after surgery in the extremities (fractures, arthroplasties). They were used immediately after surgery for a week. Some of the observed benefits include milder and fewer postoperative complications, improved blood supply to the extremities, faster wound healing, and the positive attitude of patients towards new therapies, which is also important. Studies conducted by American physicians from 1981 to 1984 confirmed these earlier observations, and also proved that the time of hospitalization of patients with CPM therapy was shorter compared to the control group, which used traditional rehabilitation. A number of devices have been constructed for CPM, including American devices, called Auto-Flex, the Toronto Medical Corporation's CPM, the German Artromot, and the Chinese or Italian Physiotek or Canwell. They allow the performance of physiological motions in the joints in a certain direction (depending on the device) and predetermined range of motion. At the same time it is possible to adjust the size of the leverage individually to the patient's posture, so that movements are performed in accordance with the joint axes. The authors of studies of the impact of CPM on the musculo-skeletal system draw attention to improved metabolism within the exercised joints, accelerated wound healing, decreasing periarticular soft tissue tension, more rapid absorption of the intra-articular hematoma, better blood supply to the limb, increased strength in the ligaments, and the antiedema and antithrombotic effects and lack of pain during exercise, thus hastening patient recovery (O'Driscoll & Giori, 2000).

6.2 Devices with biofeedback

One of the methods currently used in rehabilitation after total hip and knee replacement is the use of devices with biological feedback (biofeedback). These include visual feedback (in the form of images, charts, colors), auditory (sounds of changing intensity), thermal and strength biofeedback. The patient, thanks to the information obtained about how to perform a specific task (depending on the device used) can constantly and actively alter the force required for its implementation, or the method, or the direction, for example, so as to achieve the desired level of accuracy. Treatment with biofeedback is especially helpful in patients with locomotor pathology, which results in disorders in the control of movements, the formation of abnormal movement patterns or problems with balance. Among pathological process of this type, degenerative arthritis of the lower limbs and its surgical treatment can undoubtedly be included, since these disorders lead to disturbances in the normal gait model. Gradual progressive restriction of motion and increasing pain often cause severe impairment of both the mechanics and efficiency of gait. It is not uncommon for patients who have had degenerative arthritis for many years to move with crutches or a cane, and their gait causes pain and becomes increasingly more tiring. Arthroplasty and the postoperative period are also associated with different types of gait disorders, which may also lead to a shift in the center of gravity, which in turn causes an overload of other structures of the musculoskeletal system. Incorrect motor habits often become fixed. It is important, then, after arthroplasty, either hip or knee, for the rehabilitation program to include gait re-education, which can be supported by exercises using biofeedback to restore normal movement patterns (Kuczma et al., 2007; Rasch et al., 2010; Wilk-Frańczuk et al., 2010).

Many types of devices using biological feedback are currently available. Among these are static-dynamic parapodia, which, through dedicated computer software, use mostly video and audio feedback. This allows for balance exercises involving, for example, appropriate balancing and moving the center of gravity, with a visual record of the results. Through these exercises the patient learns to consciously control a particular function in a manner adequate to received visual and auditory information. Parapodia are also used to achieve a passive standing position from sitting in a wheelchair or a chair, while enabling the patient to control the speed of standing up. Another type of device is a gyro, some of which are controlled by computer-aided motion with the possibility of using an electric motor drive. They allow for exercises against active or passive resistance, with a capacity for resistance grading. Visual feedback of speed and asymmetry of the lower limbs are used for this purpose. These rotors are used, among other things, for gait re-education, in order to mitigate the consequences of limitations of physical activity in people with weak muscle strength and spasms. After each exercise the computer built into the device displays an analysis of the training just completed.

Studies on the suitability of equipment using biofeedback show that they allow for the confirmation of function improvement, control of distribution of weight, and stronger patient motivation to take on new tasks related to functional improvement.

6.3 Cryotherapy

Cryotherapy, or surface application of cryogenic temperatures to trigger the body's physiological response to cold, can be applied in various forms. It is primarily local cryotherapy that is used, by means of a device that employs liquid nitrogen, carbon dioxide or chilled air. Another form of cryotherapy, general cryotherapy, involves subjecting the patient's whole body to the effects of low temperatures (-110°C - -160°C) in a cryochamber. In the case of local cryotherapy, the lowest temperatures (measured at the outlet of the nozzle) are obtained by using liquid nitrogen. Cryotherapy is used in many diseases, including ankylosing spondylitis, rheumatoid arthritis (RA), degenerative joint disease, overstrain and traumatic diseases of the musculoskeletal system, or in persistent pain syndromes. Many authors have shown a positive effect on pain reduction, an anti-inflammatory effect, an antiedema effect, and reduced muscle tension. Low temperatures, thanks to the body's physiological reactions, also make it possible to intensify kinesitherapy. In most patients, the use of topical cooling at very low temperatures results in subjectively pleasurable sensations. This is mainly due to the abolition of pain, enabling intensive exercise, which leads in turn to improved joint mobility sufficient to perform basic activities free of pain. Local cryotherapy treatment implemented in the rehabilitation protocol reduces pain in all patients after total knee replacement, reduces or eliminates edema of the operated lower extremity, and by its analgesic and antiedema effect improves gait efficiency and esthetics. Cryotherapy treatment in the vicinity of the knee allows the cooling of this area of the body by about 10°C, followed by the application of kinesitherapy to speed up warming of the tissues, so that after about 15 minutes the temperature approaches the baseline temperature. Patients with no kinesitherapy after local cryotherapy around the knee note slower warming of the same area (Wilk et al., 2008). The observed effect of faster return of temperature to the baseline value may be due to the so-called after-effect phenomenon, consisting in the fact that intra-articular temperature is close to skin temperature and, unlike the muscles, under the influence of the cessation of cooling is not further reduced. Thus cryotherapy treatments performed on joints require direct kinesitherapy afterwards in order to make proper use the effect of cryotherapy, as was confirmed in the study (Wilk & Frańczuk, 2005b; Wilk et al., 2008).

7. References

Będziński, R. & Ścigała, K. (2000). Biomechanika stawu biodrowego i kolanowego. In. Biocybernetyka i Inżynieria Biomedyczna 2000. Tom 5. Nałęcz M. (Ed.), pp.113-158. EXIT ISSN 83-87674-67-2, Warszawa, Poland

Burnfield, J.M., Shu, Y., Buster, T. & Taylor, A. (2010). Similarity of Joint Kinematics and Muscle Demands Between Eliptical Training and Walking: Implication for Practice. *Physical Therapy*, Vol.90, No. 2, pp. 289-305, p-ISSN 0031-9023, e-ISSN 1538-6724

Cichy, B. & Wilk, M. (2006) Gait analysis in osteoarthritis of the hip. *Medical Science Monitor*, Vol. 12, No. 12, pp. 507-513. p-ISSN 1234-1010, e-ISSN 1634-3750

Cichy, B., Wilk, M. & Śliwiński, Z. (2008). Changes in gait parameters in total hip arthroplasty patients before and after surgery. *Medical Science Monitor*, Vol. 14, No. 3, pp. 159-169, p-ISSN 1234-1010, e-ISSN 1634-3750

Dudda, M., Gueleryuez, A., Gautier, E., Busato, A. & Roeder, C. (2010). Risk factors for early dislocation after total hip arthroplasty: a matched case-control study. *Journal of Orthopaedic Surgery*, Vol. 18, No. 2, pp. 179-183, ISSN 1022-5536

Evgeniadis, G., Beneka, A., Malliou, P., Mavromoustakos, S. & Godolias, G. (2008). Effects of pre- or postoperative therapeutic exercise on the quality of life, before and after total knee arthroplasty for osteoarthritis. *Journal of Back and Musculoskeletal Rehabilitation*, No. 21, pp. 161–169, ISSN 1053-8127

Giaquinto, S., Ciotola, E., Margutti, F. & Valentini, F. (2007). Gait during hydrokinesitherapy following total hip arthroplasty. *Disability and Rehabilitation*, Vol. 29, No. 9, pp. 743 – 749, ISSN 0963-8288

Grotle, M., Garratt, A.M., Klokkerud, M., Løchting, I., Uhlig, T. & Hagen, T.B. (2010). What's in Team Rehabilitation Care After Arthroplasty for Osteoarthritis? Results From a Multicenter, Longitudinal Study Assessing Structure, Process, and Outcome. *Physical Therapy*, Vol. 90, No. 1, pp. 121-131, p-ISSN 0031-9023, e-ISSN 1538-6724

Iyengar, K.P., Nadkarni, J.B., Ivanovic, N. & Mahale, A. (2007). Targeted early rehabilitation at home after total hip and knee joint replacement: Does it work?. *Disability and Rehabilitation*, Vol. 29, No. 6, pp. 495-502, ISSN 0963-8288

Kabsch, A. & Bober, T. (2001). Selected issues in the biomechanics of the knee joint. *Polish Journal of Physiotherapy*, Vol. 1, No. 2, pp. 179-182, ISSN 1642-0136

Kuczma, W., Srokowska, A., Owczarzak, M., Hoffman, J., Hagner, W. & Srokowski, G. (2007). The Phenomenon of Biofeedback in Neurological Rehabilitation Traded on "Balance Trainer". *Acta Balneologica*, Vol. 49, No. 2, pp. 79-85, ISSN 0005-4202

Maguire, C., Sieben, J.M., Frank, M., & Romkes, J. (2010). Hip abductor control in walking following stroke – the immediate effect of canes, taping and TheraTogs on gait. *Clinical Rehabilitation*, No. 24, pp. 37–45, p-ISSN 0269-2155, e-ISSN 1477-0873

Marks, R. (2010). Disabling hip osteoarthritis: gender, body mass, health and functional status correlates. *Health*, Vol. 7, No. 2, pp. 696-704, ISSN 1949-4998

Moody, J. (2000). Recommendations for the medical management of osteoarthritis of the hip and knee . 2000 Update American College of Rheumatology Subcommittee on Osteoarthritis Guidelines. *Arthritis & Rheumatism*, No .43, pp. 1905-1915, ISSN 0004-3591

Nolewajka, M., Gaździk, Sz.& Wieczorek, P. (2008). DVT risk factors after Total hip or knee replacement. *Journal of Orthoppaedics Trauma Surgery and Related Research*, Vol. 3, No. 11, pp. 17-30, ISSN 1897-2276

O'Driscoll, S.W. & Giori, N.J. (2000). Continuous passive motion (CPM): Theory and principles of clinical application. *Journal Res. & Dev*, Vol. 37, No. 2, pp. 179-188.

Piva, S.R., Teixeira, P.E.P., Almeida, G.J.M., Gil, A.B., DiGioia, III A.M., Levison, T.J. & Fitzgerald G.K. (2011). Contribution of Hip Abductor Strength to Physical Function in Patients With Total Knee Arthroplasty. *Physical Therapy*, Vol. 91, No.2, pp. 225-233. p-ISSN 0031-9023, e-ISSN 1538-6724

Rasch, A., Dalén, N. & Berg, H.E. (2010). Muscle strength, gait, and balance in 20 patients with hip osteoarthritis followed for 2 years after THA. *Acta Orthopaedica*, Vol. 81, No. 2, pp. 183–188, ISSN 1745-3674

Starowicz, A., Szwarczyk, W., Wilk, M. & Frańczuk, B. (2005). The evaluation of quality of life among patients after total hip replacement. *Polish Journal of Physiotherapy*, Vol. 5, No. 3, pp. 313-322, ISSN 1642-0136

Wilk, M. & Frańczuk, B. (2003). Analysis of changes in the strenght of muscles acting on the hip joint in patients recovering from hip arthroplasty. *Polish Journal of Physiotherapy*, Vol. 3, No. 4, pp. 309-315, ISSN 1642-0136

Wilk, M. & Frańczuk, B. (2004). Evaluating changes in the range of movement in the hip joint in patients with degenerative changes, before and after total hip replacement. *Ortopedia Traumatologia Rehabilitacja*, Vol. 6, No. 3, pp. 342-349, ISSN 1509-3492

Wilk, M. & Frańczuk, B. (2005a). Rehabilitation of patients after hip arthroplasty using Continuous Passive Motion. *Polish Journal of Physiotherapy*, Vol. 5, No. 1, pp. 8-14, ISSN 1642-0136

Wilk, M. & Frańczuk, B. (2005b). Local cryotherapy in patients recovering from total knee replacement. *Polish Journal of Physiotherapy*, Vol. 5, No. 3, pp. 329-333, ISSN 1642-0136

Wilk, M., Frańczuk, B., Trąbka, R. & Szwarczyk, W. (2004). Outcome of early rehabilitation with continuous passive motion for patients recovering from surgical reconstruction of the knee due to degenerative changes. A preliminary report. *Polish Journal of Physiotherapy*, Vol. 4, No. 2, pp. 163-166, ISSN 1642-0136

Wilk, M., Trąbka, R. & Śliwiński, Z. (2008). Changes in knee joint thermograms following local cryotherapy combined with various physiotherapy regimens. *Polish Journal of Physiotherapy*, Vol. 8, No 3, pp. 267-271, ISSN 1642-0136

Wilk-Frańczuk, M., Tomaszewski, W., Zemła, J., Noga, H. & Czamara, A. (2011). Analysis of rehabilitation procedure following arthroplasty of the knee with the use of complete endoprosthesis. *Medical Science Monitor*, Vol. 17, No. 3, pp. 165-168, p-ISSN 1234-1010, e-ISSN 1634-3750

Wilk-Frańczuk, M., Zemła, J. & Śliwiński, Z. (2010). The application of biofeedback exercises in patients following arthroplasty of the knee with the use of total endoprothesis. *Medical Science Monitor*, Vol. 16, No. 9, pp. 423-426, p-ISSN 1234-1010, e-ISSN 1634-3750

Wright, A.A., Cook, C.E., Flynn, T.W., Baxter, G.D. & Abbott, J.H. (2011). Predictors of Response to Physical Therapy Intervention in Patients With Primary Hip Osteoarthritis. *Physical Therapy*, Vol. 91, No. 4, pp. 510-524, p-ISSN 0031-9023, e-ISSN 1538-6724

Zeni, Jr J.A. & Snyder-Mackler, L. (2010). Early Postoperative Measures Predict 1- and 2-Year Outcomes After Unilateral Total Knee Arthroplasty: Importance of Contralateral Limb Strength. *Physical Therapy*, Vol. 90, No. 1, pp. 43-54, p-ISSN 0031-9023, e-ISSN 1538-6724

Part 2

Special Topics in Hip Arthroplasty

9

Surface Replacement of Hip Joint

Hiran Amarasekera and Damian Griffin
*1Orthopaedic Research Fellow/PhD Student, Warwick Orthopaedics
University of Warwick Medical School
2Professor of Trauma and Orthopaedics, Warwick Orthopaedics
University of Warwick Medical School
United Kingdom*

1. Introduction

Surface hip replacement more commonly known as hip resurfacing arthroplasty is a type of a hip replacement that is different to a total hip replacement. In a total hip replacement femoral head and neck are removed and a metal stem is inserted to the femoral shaft. In hip resurfacing articular surface is shaved and a metal cap (Fig 1) is inserted preserving most of the bone in femoral head and neck.

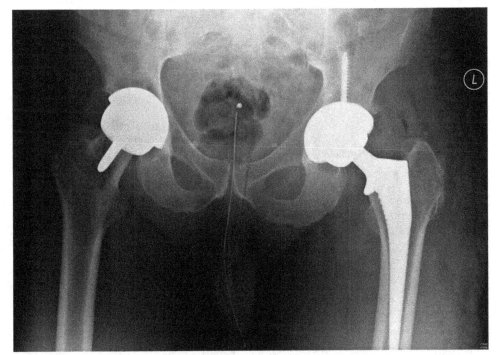

Fig. 1. X Ray shows a Hip Resurfacing arthroplasty (Right) and a Total Hip Replacement (Left)

Compared to the total hip replacement resurfacing arthroplasty preserves more bone on the femoral side (Fig.1). Acetabular replacement is similar to both procedures. Main advantages of surface replacement include preservation of femoral bone stock; increase degree of motion, and easier conversion to a total hip replacement during revision. All these make resurfacing arthroplasty an attractive alternative to a total hip replacement especially in the young active adults.

2. History

Professor Sir John in initially introduced hip resurfacing early in 1950s. (Charnley 1960; McMinn and Daniel 2006) The initial designs were uncemented PTFE (polytetrafluaroethelene) on metal. All early implants had an acetabular component made of softer material such as PFFE and femoral component made of metal. This combination of hard on soft surface caused many problems.
The previous designs failed due to two main reasons. Firstly combination of hard on soft surfaces and large diameter heads lead to increase wear, wear particle accumulation, osteolysis of the bone.
Secondly posterior approach used during the procedure damaged the blood supply to the femoral head. This lead to reduced femoral head vascularity, osteonecrosis, femoral neck fractures, and aseptic loosening of the implant.
Due to these problems hip resurfacings in the 50s through 80s were not a popular option to treat arthritis in the young adult. However in early 1990s *McMinn et al (McMinn et al. 1996)* introduced the modern hip resurfacing which used metal on metal bearings with improved instrumentation for precision placement of implants. It was believed metal on metal reduce the wear and tear of the implanted hip. Vascularity too was addressed by proposing many surgical approaches such as the trochanteric flip(Ganz et al. 2001) antero-lateral(Jacobs, Goytia, and Bhargava 2008) or direct-lateral (Hardinge 1982)as alternative approaches to the conventional posterior approach which is widely used in total hip replacement.
Hip resurfacings has been conducted in many centres since early 1990 as popular option in treating young active adults with hip problems. However with time long term results from the modern surface replacements has identified it's own set of complications(Shimmin, Bare, and Back 2005) such as femoral neck fractures aseptic loosening, avascular necrosis, osteolysis of head and increase metal ions levels.(Hing, Back, and Shimmin 2007)
Due to these factors the selection criteria for surface replacement has changed from a much broader set to a narrow and a limited set, over the last decade.(Nunley, Della Valle, and Barrack 2009)
At present even-though the selection criteria is narrowed it sill remains a key alternative to the conventional hip replacements.

3. Indications for hip resurfacing

When surface replacement was re introduced in early 1990 s the ideal candidate for the procedure was a young active adult with good hip morphology and a reasonably good bone quality, with osteoarthritis of the hip.(McMinn et al. 2011)

With a high range of motion and a low dislocation rate surface replacement seem to be the ideal option for a young adult who could have a near normal range of motion following resurfacing arthroplasty. If the patient requires a revision to total hip replacement then this could be delayed and a second revision delayed even further. As people live longer with an increasing life expectancy rate this enables the orthopaedic surgeon to delay the first total hip replacement. (Della Valle, Nunley, and Barrack 2008; Hing, Back, and Shimmin 2007)

However with the availability of the long-term complications of hip resurfacing arthroplasty the initial interest that prevailed in early 1990s has waned over the last few years and, many surgeons have narrowed selection criteria down.

3.1 Selection criteria
3.1.1 Age
55 years for women 65 years for men.(Corten et al. 2011)

3.1.2 Sex
Resurfacing is better tolerated by men than women. Pre-menopausal women have a better chance than the post menopausal women as the femoral neck fracture rate increases after menopause.(Shimmin and Back 2005) Some studies suggest that surgical technique, implant selection, and implant positioning should be modified according to the gender. If this is done there is a high possibility that gender specific bias can be eliminated, as this is a common problem in surface replacement.(Amstutz, Wisk, and Le Duff 2011; Jameson et al. 2008)

3.1.3 Pathology of the hip
Ideal candidate for a hip resurfacing is a patient with primary osteoarthritis. However most patients do not develop primary osteoarthritis at an early age. Younger patients developing osteoarthritis is mostly due to secondary causes. Surface replacement of the hip has been performed in many pathological conditions that eventually lead to secondary osteoarthritis. However conditions in which the bone may be weak such as osteoporosis, resurfacings should be avoided as this can lead to high incidence of femoral neck fractures. Avascular necrosis (AVN) is a relative contraindication for hip resurfacing. Even though some surgeons have performed hip resurfacing in AVN patients most surgeons believe that resurfacing should not be done on these patients. Partial hip resurfacing/hemi resurfacing seems to be the popular treatment option for patients with Avascular Necrosis. In partial resurfacing only the necrotic area of the articular surface is removed and replaced (Fig 2).(Siguier et al. 2001; Ushio et al. 2003) Partial resurfacing is also done for localised osteochondral defects. (Van Stralen et al. 2009)

The indications for hip resurfacing has changed during the past decade as high failure rates were observed among certain patient groups.(McMinn et al. 2011)

This has lead to a re think and development of more stringent patient selection criteria.

3.2 Surgical techniques
Surgical approach to the hip is similar to the approaches done when performing a total hip replacement. However there are many additional considerations to be kept in mind when

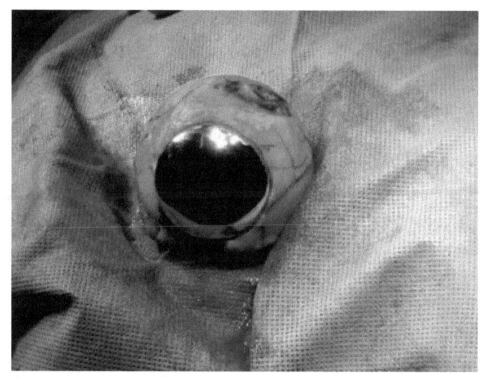

Fig. 2. Partial resurfacing done on a patient with an osteochondral defect

performing a resurfacing arthroplasty. As more bone is preserved in femoral head and the neck preserving the vascularity is a key issue. (McBryde et al. 2008) Therefore some surgeons do not use the traditional posterior approach when performing a hip resurfacing. This is because the posterior approach cuts the medial circumflex femoral artery (MCFA) main artery supplying of the femoral head and neck. This damage is believed to cause AVN of femoral head. Most studies demonstrated a fall in blood supply during posterior approach compared to other surgical approaches.(Beaule, Campbell, and Shim 2006; Bradley, Freeman, and Revell 1987; Howie, Cornish, and Vernon-Roberts 1993) However some authors including us have questioned the clinical significance of this drop as we are not clear whether the drop is transient or permanent and whether it is below the critical ischaemic level to cause the death of osteocytes in the femoral head.(Amarasekera et al. 2008)

Common alternative approach that is described to preserve blood flow was described by *Ganz et al* as the trochanteric flip approach.(Ganz et al. 2001) This is an anterior type of approach done by doing a trochanteric flip osteotomy. This approach preserves the MCFA and the main blood supply to the femoral head. Therefore it is believed in theory that the vascularity is better preserved by this approach as compared to the posterior approach. However the key disadvantage of this approach is that the patient has to be non weight bearing for four to six weeks until the trochanteric flip osteotomy heals. The other approaches describe for resurfacing include(Gerdesmeyer et al. 2008) antero lateral approach, direct lateral approach(Hardinge 1982), and minimally invasive approaches. (McMinn et al. 2005; Mont, Ragland, and Marker 2005)

Studies have been done not only to evaluate intra-operative (Amarasekera et al. 2008) as well as post-operative blood supply (Forrest et al. 2006) following different surgical approaches in resurfacing arthroplasty patients.

Post-operative vascularity has been studied using SPECT (Single Positron Emission Computed Tomography) scanning. The attenuation factor affecting the accuracy of the results in the presence of metal implants has been addressed by performing phantom studies. (Amarasekera et al. 2011)

Once a suitable surgical approach is chosen the next steps in the surgery are fairly straightforward. The acetabular replacement is similar to a THR. However the femoral head replacement is far more a demanding task as the placement of the cup is crucial and needs accuracy. This is a technically demanding procedure compared to a placing the femoral component in a THR. Poorly positioned components will lead to high wear rates, impingement and dislocations. Due to the technically demanding nature of the procedure training surgeons is challenging and has a to slow learning curve.(Berend et al. 2011) Due to this using navigation to position implants has been tried but does not appear to have an advantage over the learning curve.(Saithna and Dekker 2009; Shields et al. 2009)

To cement or not to cement the implants is another point that has been debated over the years.

When surface replacements were re introduced most implants were cemented. Therefore cementing technique and the type of cement used, area of the component cemented, all seem to contribute to the success of surgery.(Bitsch and Schmalzried 2008; Bitsch et al. 2008) Specific cementing techniques have been described when cementing the femoral component. (Bitsch et al. 2008; Bitsch et al. 2007; Chandler et al. 2006) Achieving the correct cement mantle is a technically challenging procedure. Too much cement can cause thermal necrosis while too little cement can cause a poor penetration and femoral loosening where as an extreme thin mantle can cause mechanical failure leading to high wear particles further leading to osteolysis.(Scheerlinck, Delport, and Kiewitt 2010)

Due to these controversies some surgeons adapt partially cementing the component avoiding the pin, (Schlegel et al. 2011) and some surgeons have totally stopped using cement. This lead to development of uncemented hip resurfacings and has become the procedure of choice among some surgeons.

4. Complications of surface replacements

It is worth mentioning that all general complications associated with hip surgery such as infection, bleeding, DVT, are seen with hip resurfacings. Apart from these there is a set of complications that is unique to this procedure. These are outlined below.

4.1 Avascular necrosis of femoral head (Bradley, Freeman, and Revell 1987; Little et al. 2005)

As described earlier avascular necrosis of the femoral head and neck is a potential complication that can result in failure of the implant. The main reason for this is the damage to blood supply that occurs during posterior approach. (Amarasekera et al. 2008)Avoiding posterior approach and adapting other approaches such as antero-lateral or trochanteric flip approaches(Ganz et al. 2001, 2001) will minimise this.

4.2 Femoral neck fractures

This is a known complication that can range between 0- up to1.8% after hip resurfacing.(Steffen et al. 2009) Avascular necrosis(Steffen et al. 2010), mechanical factors such as notching, femoral neck lengthening, and varus mal alignment of the femoral component has been attributed as contributory causes for femoral neck fractures.. Some studies suggest females (3%) have a higher incidence than males (1.3%) (Jameson et al. 2008) while other studies do not find any difference between the sexes.(Steffen et al. 2009) Failure rate and revision rate too seem to be higher in females as compared to males.(Carrothers et al. 2010)

4.3 Aseptic loosening of components, osteolysis, pseudo tumours, and ALVAL (Aseptic Lymphocytic Vasculitis Associated Lesions), (Zustin et al. 2009)

Large head size in hip resurfacing causes increase wear and tear leading to high metal particles. Some escape to blood flow causing high metal ion levels in blood. Some trigger an immune response leading to metallosis, aseptic loosening, lymphocytic infiltration, and osteolysis and bone resorbtion. It is less clear whether this same reaction can be triggered by cement particles. Developing a proper cementing technique(Campbell et al. 2009) or considering uncemented implants may help to minimise these complications. However dealing with increase wear metal particles remains a challenging problem.

These complications are due to series of immune reactions that occur as the body respond to large number of wear particles or cement. In early sixties these were common when metal on plastic implants were used it was a major cause for failure but with metal on metal it was thought that these would be minimal.(Zustin et al. 2010) However long term results of modern hip resurfacings suggest that the problem still exists. Recent systematic review suggests aseptic loosening to be the most common complication reported in hip resurfacing.(van der Weegen et al. 2011) (Zustin et al. 2009)

4.4 Persistent groin pain (Bin Nasser et al. 2010; Bartelt et al. 2010; Campbell et al. 2008; Nikolaou et al. 2009) and femoroacetabular impingement(Lim et al. 2011; Yoo et al. 2011)

These are mainly caused by mechanical problems such as poor positioning of implants. (Bin Nasser et al. 2010)

Carrothers et al reported prevalence of complications following surface replacement of 5000 hips in a multi surgeon series involving 141 surgeons.(Carrothers et al. 2010)These are given below (Table 1)

Complication	Number of hips	Prevalence
Fracture Neck of femur	54	1.1%
Loosening -Acetabular	32	0.6%
Femoral head AVN	30	0.6%
Loosening-Femoral	19	0.4%
Infection	17	0.3%
ALVAL/Metallosis	15	0.3%
Loosening-Both	05	0.1%
Dislocation	05	0.1%
Revision rate	182	3.6%

Table 1. Complications reported by *Carrothers et al*

5. Conclusion

When resurface was first done initial complications were due to high wear between metal and plastic surface. This is because the surface area of the resurfacing femoral head is much larger that the surface area of a THR implant. This causes more frictional forces between the acetabular and femoral components producing increase wear particles. When the head was metal and the cup was plastic the wear rate was even higher and this lead to initially failure of the original designs. To avoid this problem the modern implants were designed as metal on metal expecting the wear to be a less significant. Recent evidence suggest collection of metal particles within the tissues causes metallosis and leaking metal to the blood stream has caused high metal ion levels, (Clarke et al. 2003; Vendittoli et al. 2010; Vendittoli, Ganapathi, and Lavigne 2007)metal allergies, and metallosis. This has been attributed to triggering immunological reactions such as ALVAL, Pseudo tumour formations, resorbtion of head finally leading to loosening and implant failure.

Due to all these complications resurfacing arthroplasty has fallen out of favour as the automatic procedure of choice to treat young active patient with hip problems.

This has re opened the debate on how best to treat young active adults with hip problems. Uncemented hip replacement, minimal invasive techniques, and arthroscopic hip procedures are a few options that should be considered as an alternative to hip resurfacing in selected patients.

Nevertheless surface replacement done on a carefully selected patient by a highly trained surgeon taking in to consideration the surgical approach, cementing technique, implant selection and implant positioning will increase the success rate of the procedure.

6. References

Amarasekera, H. W., M. L. Costa, P. Foguet, S. J. Krikler, U. Prakash, and D. R. Griffin. 2008. The blood flow to the femoral head/neck junction during resurfacing arthroplasty: A COMPARISON OF TWO APPROACHES USING LASER DOPPLER FLOWMETRY. *J Bone Joint Surg Br* 90 (4):442-5.

Amarasekera, H. W., M. L. Costa, N. Parsons, J. Achten, D. R. Griffin, S. Manktelow, and N. R. Williams. 2011. SPECT/CT bone imaging after hip resurfacing arthroplasty: is it feasible to use CT attenuation correction in the presence of metal implants? *Nucl Med Commun* 32 (4):289-97.

Amstutz, H. C., L. E. Wisk, and M. J. Le Duff. 2011. Sex as a patient selection criterion for metal-on-metal hip resurfacing arthroplasty. *J Arthroplasty* 26 (2):198-208.

Bartelt, R. B., B. J. Yuan, R. T. Trousdale, and R. J. Sierra. 2010. The prevalence of groin pain after metal-on-metal total hip arthroplasty and total hip resurfacing. *Clin Orthop Relat Res* 468 (9):2346-56.

Beaule, P. E., P. Campbell, and P. Shim. 2006. Femoral Head Blood Flow during Hip Resurfacing. *Clin Orthop Relat Res.*

Berend, K. R., A. V. Lombardi, Jr., J. B. Adams, and M. A. Sneller. 2011. Unsatisfactory surgical learning curve with hip resurfacing. *J Bone Joint Surg Am* 93 Suppl 2:89-92.

Bin Nasser, A., P. E. Beaule, M. O'Neill, P. R. Kim, and A. Fazekas. 2010. Incidence of groin pain after metal-on-metal hip resurfacing. *Clin Orthop Relat Res* 468 (2):392-9.

Bitsch, R. G., C. Heisel, M. Silva, and T. P. Schmalzried. 2007. Femoral cementing technique for hip resurfacing arthroplasty. *J Orthop Res* 25 (4):423-31.

Bitsch, R. G., T. Loidolt, C. Heisel, and T. P. Schmalzried. 2008. Cementing techniques for hip resurfacing arthroplasty: development of a laboratory model. *J Bone Joint Surg Am* 90 Suppl 3:102-10.

Bitsch, R. G., and T. P. Schmalzried. 2008. [Cementing techniques for hip resurfacing arthroplasty. What do we know?]. *Orthopade* 37 (7):667-71.

Bradley, G. W., M. A. Freeman, and P. A. Revell. 1987. Resurfacing arthroplasty. Femoral head viability. *Clin Orthop Relat Res* (220):137-41.

Campbell, P., A. Shimmin, L. Walter, and M. Solomon. 2008. Metal sensitivity as a cause of groin pain in metal-on-metal hip resurfacing. *J Arthroplasty* 23 (7):1080-5.

Campbell, P., K. Takamura, W. Lundergan, C. Esposito, and H. C. Amstutz. 2009. Cement technique changes improved hip resurfacing longevity - implant retrieval findings. *Bull NYU Hosp Jt Dis* 67 (2):146-53.

Carrothers, A. D., R. E. Gilbert, A. Jaiswal, and J. B. Richardson. 2010. Birmingham hip resurfacing: the prevalence of failure. *J Bone Joint Surg Br* 92 (10):1344-50.

Chandler, M., R. S. Kowalski, N. D. Watkins, A. Briscoe, and A. M. New. 2006. Cementing techniques in hip resurfacing. *Proc Inst Mech Eng H* 220 (2):321-31.

Charnley, J. 1960. Surgery of the hip-joint: present and future developments. *Br Med J* 1 (5176):821-6.

Clarke, M. T., P. T. Lee, A. Arora, and R. N. Villar. 2003. Levels of metal ions after small- and large-diameter metal-on-metal hip arthroplasty. *J Bone Joint Surg Br* 85 (6):913-7.

Corten, K., R. Ganz, J. P. Simon, and M. Leunig. 2011. Hip resurfacing arthroplasty: current status and future perspectives. *Eur Cell Mater* 21:243-58.

Della Valle, C. J., R. M. Nunley, and R. L. Barrack. 2008. When is the right time to resurface? *Orthopedics* 31 (12 Suppl 2).

Forrest, N., A. Welch, A. D. Murray, L. Schweiger, J. Hutchison, and G. P. Ashcroft. 2006. Femoral head viability after Birmingham resurfacing hip arthroplasty: assessment with use of [18F] fluoride positron emission tomography. *J Bone Joint Surg Am* 88 Suppl 3:84-9.

Ganz, R., T. J. Gill, E. Gautier, K. Ganz, N. Krugel, and U. Berlemann. 2001. Surgical dislocation of the adult hip a technique with full access to the femoral head and acetabulum without the risk of avascular necrosis. *J Bone Joint Surg Br* 83 (8):1119-24.

— — —. 2001. Surgical dislocation of the adult hip: A TECHNIQUE WITH FULL ACCESS TO THE FEMORAL HEAD AND ACETABULUM WITHOUT THE RISK OF AVASCULAR NECROSIS. *J Bone Joint Surg Br* 83-B (8):1119-1124.

Gerdesmeyer, L., H. Gollwitzer, R. Bader, and M. Rudert. 2008. [Surgical approaches in hip resurfacing]. *Orthopade* 37 (7):650-8.

Hardinge, K. 1982. The direct lateral approach to the hip. *J Bone Joint Surg Br* 64 (1):17-9.

Hing, C., D. Back, and A. Shimmin. 2007. Hip resurfacing: indications, results, and conclusions. *Instr Course Lect* 56:171-8.

Howie, D. W., B. L. Cornish, and B. Vernon-Roberts. 1993. The viability of the femoral head after resurfacing hip arthroplasty in humans. *Clin Orthop Relat Res* (291):171-84.

Jacobs, M. A., R. N. Goytia, and T. Bhargava. 2008. Hip resurfacing through an anterolateral approach. Surgical description and early review. *J Bone Joint Surg Am* 90 Suppl 3:38-44.

Jameson, S. S., D. J. Langton, S. Natu, and T. V. Nargol. 2008. The influence of age and sex on early clinical results after hip resurfacing: an independent center analysis. *J Arthroplasty* 23 (6 Suppl 1):50-5.

Lim, S. J., J. H. Kim, Y. W. Moon, and Y. S. Park. 2011. Femoroacetabular Cup Impingement After Resurfacing Arthroplasty of the Hip. *J Arthroplasty*.

Little, C. P., A. L. Ruiz, I. J. Harding, P. McLardy-Smith, R. Gundle, D. W. Murray, and N. A. Athanasou. 2005. Osteonecrosis in retrieved femoral heads after failed resurfacing arthroplasty of the hip. *J Bone Joint Surg Br* 87 (3):320-3.

McBryde, C. W., M. P. Revell, A. M. Thomas, R. B. Treacy, and P. B. Pynsent. 2008. The influence of surgical approach on outcome in Birmingham hip resurfacing. *Clin Orthop Relat Res* 466 (4):920-6.

McMinn, D., and J. Daniel. 2006. History and modern concepts in surface replacement. *Proc Inst Mech Eng H* 220 (2):239-51.

McMinn, D. J., J. Daniel, P. B. Pynsent, and C. Pradhan. 2005. Mini-incision resurfacing arthroplasty of hip through the posterior approach. *Clin Orthop Relat Res* 441:91-8.

McMinn, D. J., J. Daniel, H. Ziaee, and C. Pradhan. 2011. Indications and results of hip resurfacing. *Int Orthop* 35 (2):231-7.

McMinn, D., R. Treacy, K. Lin, and P. Pynsent. 1996. Metal on metal surface replacement of the hip. Experience of the McMinn prothesis. *Clin Orthop Relat Res* (329 Suppl):S89-98.

Mont, M. A., P. S. Ragland, and D. Marker. 2005. Resurfacing hip arthroplasty: comparison of a minimally invasive versus standard approach. *Clin Orthop Relat Res* 441:125-31.

Nikolaou, V., S. G. Bergeron, O. L. Huk, D. J. Zukor, and J. Antoniou. 2009. Evaluation of persistent pain after hip resurfacing. *Bull NYU Hosp Jt Dis* 67 (2):168-72.

Nunley, R. M., C. J. Della Valle, and R. L. Barrack. 2009. Is patient selection important for hip resurfacing? *Clin Orthop Relat Res* 467 (1):56-65.

Saithna, A., and A. P. Dekker. 2009. The influence of computer navigation on trainee learning in hip resurfacing arthroplasty. *Comput Aided Surg* 14 (4-6):117-22.

Scheerlinck, T., H. Delport, and T. Kiewitt. 2010. Influence of the cementing technique on the cement mantle in hip resurfacing: an in vitro computed tomography scan-based analysis. *J Bone Joint Surg Am* 92 (2):375-87.

Schlegel, U. J., J. Siewe, R. G. Bitsch, J. Koebke, P. Eysel, and M. M. Morlock. 2011. Influence of cementing the pin on resistance to fracture in hip resurfacing. *Clin Biomech (Bristol, Avon)* 26 (2):136-40.

Shields, J. S., T. M. Seyler, C. Maguire, and R. H. Jinnah. 2009. Computer-assisted navigation in hip resurfacing arthroplasty - a single-surgeon experience. *Bull NYU Hosp Jt Dis* 67 (2):164-7.

Shimmin, A. J., and D. Back. 2005. Femoral neck fractures following Birmingham hip resurfacing: a national review of 50 cases. *J Bone Joint Surg Br* 87 (4):463-4.

Shimmin, A. J., J. Bare, and D. L. Back. 2005. Complications associated with hip resurfacing arthroplasty. *Orthop Clin North Am* 36 (2):187-93, ix.

Siguier, T., M. Siguier, T. Judet, G. Charnley, and B. Brumpt. 2001. Partial resurfacing arthroplasty of the femoral head in avascular necrosis. Methods, indications, and results. *Clin Orthop Relat Res* (386):85-92.

Steffen, R. T., N. A. Athanasou, H. S. Gill, and D. W. Murray. 2010. Avascular necrosis associated with fracture of the femoral neck after hip resurfacing: histological assessment of femoral bone from retrieval specimens. *J Bone Joint Surg Br* 92 (6):787-93.

Steffen, R. T., P. R. Foguet, S. J. Krikler, R. Gundle, D. J. Beard, and D. W. Murray. 2009. Femoral neck fractures after hip resurfacing. *J Arthroplasty* 24 (4):614-9.

Ushio, K., M. Oka, S. H. Hyon, S. Yura, J. Toguchida, and T. Nakamura. 2003. Partial hemiarthroplasty for the treatment of osteonecrosis of the femoral head. An experimental study in the dog. *J Bone Joint Surg Br* 85 (6):922-30.

van der Weegen, W., H. J. Hoekstra, T. Sijbesma, E. Bos, E. H. Schemitsch, and R. W. Poolman. 2011. Survival of metal-on-metal hip resurfacing arthroplasty: a systematic review of the literature. *J Bone Joint Surg Br* 93 (3):298-306.

Van Stralen, R. A., D. Haverkamp, C. J. Van Bergen, and H. Eijer. 2009. Partial resurfacing with varus osteotomy for an osteochondral defect of the femoral head. *Hip Int* 19 (1):67-70.

Vendittoli, P. A., M. Ganapathi, and M. Lavigne. 2007. Blood and urine metal ion levels in young and active patients after Birmingham hip resurfacing arthroplasty. *J Bone Joint Surg Br* 89 (7):989; author reply 989-90.

Venditoli, P. A., A. Roy, S. Mottard, J. Girard, D. Lusignan, and M. Lavigne. 2010. Metal ion release from bearing wear and corrosion with 28 mm and large-diameter metal-on-metal bearing articulations: a follow-up study. *J Bone Joint Surg Br* 92 (1):12-9.

Yoo, M. C., Y. J. Cho, Y. S. Chun, and K. H. Rhyu. 2011. Impingement between the acetabular cup and the femoral neck after hip resurfacing arthroplasty. *J Bone Joint Surg Am* 93 Suppl 2:99-106.

Zustin, J., M. Amling, M. Krause, S. Breer, M. Hahn, M. M. Morlock, W. Ruther, and G. Sauter. 2009. Intraosseous lymphocytic infiltrates after hip resurfacing arthroplasty : a histopathological study on 181 retrieved femoral remnants. *Virchows Arch* 454 (5):581-8.

Zustin, J., M. Hahn, M. M. Morlock, W. Ruther, M. Amling, and G. Sauter. 2010. Femoral component loosening after hip resurfacing arthroplasty. *Skeletal Radiol* 39 (8):747-56.

10

Planning of Arthroplasty in Dysplastic Hips

Nevzat Selim Gokay[1], Alper Gokce[1], Bulent Alp[2] and Fahri Erdogan[2]
*[1]Namik Kemal University School of Medicine,
Department of Orthopaedics and Traumatology, Tekirdag
[2]Istanbul University, Cerrahpasa School of Medicine,
Department of Orthopaedics and Traumatology, Istanbul
Turkey*

1. Introduction

Hip dysplasia is one of the major conditions leading degenerative hip arthritis in early adulthood. Devolopmental insuffuciency of bony structures yields asymetric ball and socket formation, which usually associated with trophic changes and instability. Total hip joint replacement has successfull results in patients with hip dysplasia in adulthood. The major goal of the treatment is rebuilding of a new stable artificial joint with painless range of motion. There is a need of a meticulous preoperative planning assessing the anatomic severity of the pathology, which is consisted of involved bony and soft tissue components. Limb length discrepency, quality of bone stock, muscle atrophies, weakness and contractures should be evaluated before surgery. There are several classifications for assesment of acetabuar dysplasia. However, we are aware of a combined clasification or comprehensive allgorithym for assesment of all components of pathology in unisom.

Current devolopments in the field of radiology like Three Dimensional (3d) Computerized Tomography (CT) and Magnetic Resonance Imaging (MRI) allowed assesment of all component of hip dysplasia preoperatively. Metaphyseal and acetabular bone stock and structure, anteversion degrees and soft tissues has to be taken in consideration. The aim of this chapter is to review the present classifications and reported experiences on hip dysplasia and discuss the value of missing parts. The preoperative planning process were also reviewed regarding the role of modern radiologic examination techniques on current surgical and clinical applications.

2. Planning of arthroplasty in dysplastic hips

Patient selection is very importmant in the treatment of developmental dysplasia of the hip (DDH). In proper and young patients femoral or periacetabular osteotomy should be considered. Nevertheless total hip arthroplasty is often required for most of the patients with dysplasia. The major goal of the treatment is rebuilding of a new stable artificial joint with painless range of motion. To this end, there is a need of a meticulous preoperative planning assessing the anatomic severity of the pathology, which is consisted of involved bony and soft tissue component. The most important thing which should stick in our minds is the complexity of the anatomical abnormality complicating the reconstruction.

The orthopaedic surgeons should display a hard challenge to overcome these deformities. Serious hypoplasia of the acetabulum, femoral head deformity, short femoral neck, excessive anteversion of the neck, narrow and straight medullary canal, totally dislocation, limb leg discrepancy and highly placed trochanter are some of these deformities which makes the surgery difficult. Surgery may be further complicated by the effects of previously performed osteotomies. Therefore, an accurate guide is mandatory to solve this problem in the pre-operative planning.

2.1 An overlook to the basic science of congenital hip disease
Understanding of the embryological development of the hip, epidemiology, pathologic anatomy and the natural history of congenital hip disease (CDH) should help us to conceive the disease with accuracy and improve our skills in surgical area.

2.1.1 Embryology and normal development of the hip
The acetabulum and femoral head develope from the same mesenchymal cells in a cleft at the tenth week of the gestational period (Gardner & Gray, 1950; Strayer, 1943) Hip joint is completely formed at the 11th week of gestation. It is initially deeply set and spherical. It becomes progressively less deeply set and hemispherical until birth. The hip has maximum range of motion at birth as it is shallowest. They thought that this adaptation help the fetus pass through the birth canal. After birth these trends reverse : the acetabulum becomes deeper again and the femoral head more spherical. This process continues throughout childhood. Thus the risk of dislocation is greatest at the prenatal period.(Rális & McKibbin, 1973; Watanabe, 1974; Wedge & Wasylenko, 1978).

It is better to discuss about the normal postnatal development of the hip, before examining the pathologic anatomy of DDH. The outer two thirds of the acetabulum is formed by the acetabular cartilage. This complex is interposed between the ilium, the pubis and the ischium. It is rich from hyaline cartilage cells and contains growth plates on each side which helps the hip socket to expand during growth. (Ponseti, 1978; Watanabe, 1974; Weinstein, 1987). It is known that the concavity of the acetabulum develops in response to the presence of the spherical femoral head (Harrison, 1961; Smith et al., 1958).

2.1.2 Pathologic anatomy of DDH
The term of DDH was started to be used in the last decades, after it was understood that this disease presents in different manners;
1. Dysplasia: The articular relationship between femur and acetabulum isn't broken, consequently Shenton's line is intact. There is inadequate development of the acetabulum.
2. Subluxation: The femoral head migrates laterally and proximally, Shenton's line is broken but femoral head is still in contact with acetabulum.
3. Dislocation: The femoral head is completely out of the acetabulum. The displacement of the femoral head is usually in posterosuperior direction.

It seems that these are the different stages of a disease seen in ages. (Hartofilakidis et al, 2000; Weinstein, 1987)

Therefore the pathological anatomy of the disease differs in a wide spectrum and depends on the stage of the disease. The anatomical pathology in dysplasia is mostly at the acetabuler side of the joint. It is shallow than usual and femoroacetabular coverage is not enough.

This entity may cause osteoartrhritic changes and femoral head will become deformed in time. Secondary degerative changes may lead the dysplastic hip convert into a subluxed hip. In subluxation femoral head is proximally and laterally displaced. The major difference between dysplasia and subluxation is the intactness of Shenton's line on the graphies. In these cases bone stock of the acetabulum is less affected, and development of the femur is almost normal. In the otherhand, if a hip is dislocated, there is no relationship between the femoral head and acetabulum, acetabulum is too dysplasic and femoral head articulates to a false acetabulum on the iliac bone. The course of the abductor muscles changes to horizontally instead of lateral and vertical direction. The muscles also shorten in length due to the position of the trochanter major. Affected leg is shortened. Acetabulum is too much hypoplastic and the acetabular bone stock is remarkable diminished which is anteriorly. The bone stock is affected mostly in low dislocation cases due to the growth disruption of the acetabular lateral wall by the compression of the femoral head. Femur is also abnormal; it's hypoplastic, anteverted and femoral canal is narrow than usual. Capsule is elongated and thickened. The course of the nerve and arteries is altered. External rotators are elongated, also.

2.2 Land marks and classification methods of DDH

Various anatomical landmarks on conventional graphies were used to assess the degree of acetabular dysplasia. Center edge angle of Wiberg, acetabular angle of Sharp and femoral head extrusion index are some of these parameters measured using these landmarks (Heyman & Herndon, 1950; Sharp, 1961; Wiberg, 1939).

There are several classifications for the assesment of acetabular displasia. The classifications of Crowe and Hartofilakidis are the most used ones in the litarature. Crowe et al. described a method to determine degree of dysplasia in 1979 (Crowe et al., 1979). It was based on the degree of proximal femoral migration relative to the acetabulum on an anteroposterior radiograph of the pelvis. The authors differentiated the disease into four classes according to the distance between the teardrop and junction of the femoral neck and head. The amount of the proximal migration of the femoral head was measured as a percentage of the height of the femoral head or the pelvis (Table 1).

The classification of Hartofilakidis et al. classified dysplasia in three groups based on anatomic correlations (Hartofilakidis et al., 1988). The dislocated hip was described in two stages as low and high dislocation (Table 2). The other classification system, which was described by Eftekhar and Kerboul et al., was classified according to the shape of the acetabulum and head, and the side of dislocation respectively (Eftekhar, 1993; Kerboul et al., 1987). Along these most reliable ones are the classifications of Crowe and Hartofilakidis and their classifications have shown a better reproducibility than the systems of Eftekhar and Kerboul et al (Brunner et al., 2008; Decking et al., 2006). However, we are aware of a combined classification or comprehensive algorithym for assesment of all components of this pathology.

There isn't any classification available describing this disease with the all aspects of the deformity. Most of the classifications are focused on the shape and relation between the head of femur and acetabulum. Soft tissue disturbances were excluded during evaluation and the effects of this on the success of the treatment were overlooked. Transversely oriented and poorly developed abductor muscles, and shortened adductors are some of these conditions which complicates the treatment than expected. Also, none of these classifications in use considers the amount of femoral anteversion and metaphyseal development which results in discrepancy between the stem. These classifications should describe the deformity however they couldn't achieve any idea on the treatment method and the implant type.

Group	Description
I	Subluxation < 50% or proximal dislocation < 0.1% of the pelvic height
II	Subluxation 50% - 75% or proximal dislocation of 0.1% to 0.15 of pelvic height
III	Subluxation 75% - 100% or proximal dislocation of 0.15 to 0.20 of pelvic height
IV	Subluxation > 100% or proximal dislocation of > 0.20% of pelvic height

Table 1. The Classification of Crowe et al.

Type	Description
Dysplasia	The femoral head is not dislocated out of the acetabulum despite the degree of subluxation
Low Dislocation	The femoral head is dislocated and articulates with a false acetabulum which partially covers the true acetabulum to a varying degree
High Dislocation	The femoral head is dislocated and has migrated superiorly and posteriorly with no relation with any part of the true

Table 2. The Classification of Hartofilakidis et al.

2.3 The clinical presentation and indications in developmental hip disease

Most of the DDH patients have symptoms of other joints except the hip joint. The ipsilateral knee tends to be in valgus due to the hyper adductus of the hip. Low back pain may occur in patients with bilateral dislocations though to the hyperlordosis of the lumbar spine (Wedge & Wasylenko, 1978). As a result knee and lowback pain are mostly first symptoms of the disease. Most patients suffer from limping rather than the pain.

The indication of total hip prosthesis surgery in DDH, does not differ from the indications in primer arthrosis. The important point is that surgery in DDH patients is more complicated and the complication rate is higher than the others. So the indication of the surgery may be difficult in patients with minor symptoms. The main symptom for surgery indication should be the pain. Despite the complicity of the disease most of the patients of dislocation have no symptom rather than limping. It may be better to choose other treatment options in patients which have no or little pain. Limbing only, shouldn't be an indication for total hip arthroplasty.

2.4 Total hip arthroplasty surgery in DDH

Despite the advanced techniques and implants, the total hip arthroplasty in DDH still remains as a hardchallenge at the present time. The most difficult part of this challenge is to decide the best technique and optimum implant for each patient. Unfortunately there is no consensus of opinion on the surgical planning of these patients who present in a wide spectrum. The success of the operation mostly depends on the severity of the disease. According to the Crowe classification, the rate of survival at 20 years follow-up, was found as 72.7%, 70.7%, 36.7% and 15.6% for class 1,2,3 and 4, respectively (Chougle et al, 2005). Although total hip surgery is a succcessful operation in the treatment of dysplastic hips, it may present many problems due to the musculer contractures, abnormal location of the hip center, inadequate bone stock of acetabulum and femur, alterations in the hip anatomy, abductor insufficiency and leg length discrepancy (Charnley & Feagin, 1973; Hartofilakidis et al., 1996; Mulroy & Harris, 1990; Patterson & Brown, 1973; Symeonides et al., 1997).

2.4.1 The preoperative planning of DDH patients

Troelsen et al. drew our attention to the importance of the weight bearing pelvic radiographs and stated that it may allow us to determine the retroversion degree of the acetabulum more accurately (Troelsen et al., 2010). Although Standard Pelvis graphies and Judet graphies may tell us information about the acetabular osseous stock, the complicity of this disease induced the human being in searching new imaging modalities. The evolution in the imaging technologies, gives us the comfort of the understanding the pathology with all details before the surgery. CT has been used in preoperative planning and reported that important data about the morphology of the joint was obtained with the assistance of CT (Xenakis et al.,1996). 3d CT was also reported as an useful device in determining the acetabular anteversion and anterolateral deficiencies (Anda et al., 1991; Nakamura et al., 2000)

2.4.2 The exposure

Most methods of approache to the hip may be appropriate in DDH patients with slight deformity, for instance anterolateral and posterolateral exposures. Cameron et al. used Smith-Peterson approach to Crowe class 3 and 4 hips and they reported perfect results (Cameron et al., 1996). Despite their results they also reported a high rate of nerve complication. The surgical approach may be very dangerous due to the extraordinary anatomy in the highly dislocated patients. Trochanter major may serve as a good guide for the oriantation of the surgeon. Transtrochanteric or subtrochanteric aproachs are indicated for the highly dislocated patients who require retansion of the abductors. Kumar and Shair described an extended iliofemoral approach but found no advantage of this technique besides it results too much muscle dissection (Kumar & Shair, 1997).

2.4.3 The approach to the dysplastic asetabulum

It is without controversy that the approach to the acetabulum and acetabular component placement are the most important part of the reconstruction in DDH. It was reported that the osseous stock is much more at the true acetabuler area (Charnley & Feagin, 1973; Dunn

& Hess, 1976; Eftekar, 1978; Mendes et al., 1996). Though the ideal area of acetabuler component placement is thought to be the true acetabulum (Linde & Jensen, 1988; Yoder et al., 1988) and restoration of normal hip center of rotation provided good long-term results (Bozic et al., 2004; Yoder et al.,1988). The superior or lateral placement of the acetabuler cup was accused of being a risk factor for femoral and acetabuler loosening (Doehring et al., 1996; Yoder et al.,1988). Reaming the acetabulum deeply and using porous coated small acetabuler implants is usually enough to reconstruct the acetabulum. Although a lower rate of loosening has been reported in conjunction with medialization of the hip center, small prosthetic componenets require the use of a thin liner which are known to be responsible for polyethilen wear (Saikko, 1995). This is the reason that small cups are not appropriate to use in young and active patients with hip dysplasia (Dudkiewicz et al., 2002). The size of the acetabular component depends mostly on the severity of dislocation (Flecher et al., 2008). While the size of the acetabular cup used in Crowe 2 is the largest ones, smallest implants usually necesary in Crowe 4 patients. Moreover polyethylene wear found to be related to the cup inclination angle (Perka et al., 2004). Perka, also stated that there was no significant association between wear and the cup size or the thickness of the liner in their series.

The inadequate medialisation of the hip center seems to be an important factor modifying long term results (Kennedy et al., 1998; McQueary et al., 1988). The best position of the femoral head center is thought to be less than 35 mm vertically from the interteardrop line and 25 mm laterally from the teardrop (Hirakawa et al., 2001). Alternatively; controlled acetabuler medialisation (Hess & Umber, 1978; Paavilainen et al., 1990), acetabuler enlarging and bone greft augmentation (MacKenzie et al., 1996; McQueary & Johnston, 1988) or reinforcement cage reconstruction (Gill et al., 1998) are the other methods which can be used. But these techniques may lead to an excessive bone loss and the usage of long ofset femoral heads may be required.

High hip center concept was stated as an issue by Russotti (Russotti et al., 1991). They recommended to place the acetabular component at a more proximal but not more lateral position of the center of the hip in difficult acetabular reconstructions. It was stated that a longer stable fixation, than placement of the acetabular component at the true anatomical position, will be achieved if the latter approach necessitates reliance on large bulk allografts or autogenous grafts to provide most of the structural support. In a series of Dearborn et al., only 4 percent mechanical failure in 46 patients was reported after a mean of 10.4 years of follow-up duration (Dearborn et al., 1999). But, it was suggested that superior positioning of the acetabular component, leads to increased rates of loosening of the femoral and acetabular components (Pagnano, 1996). Also, Doehring reported that superolateral hip center relocation should be avoided and that superior-only relocation may be mechanically acceptable within the confines of the osseous anatomy of the acetabulum (Doehring et al, 1996). An attempt should be made to position the acetabular component in or near the true acetabular region. Hartofilakidis described the necessity of placement of the acetabuler component to the true acetabular level, in three entries; 1)The lever arm for body weight is much longer than the abductor lever arm at the level of false acetabulum and it results in an excessive load on the hip joint, 2)Shearing forces acting on the acetabular cup may lead to early loosening at the level of the false acetabulum, 3)The bone stock is usually better at the level of the true acetabulum than it is at more proximal levels ((Hartofilakidis & Karachalios, 2004). The hip center of rotation could be restored in only seventy eight (% 66) of 121 hips in a serie of Perka (Perka et al, 2004). Following the elongated capsule is often helpful in the location of the true acetabulum during surgery. However the localising of the normal hip center during the operation is not always so easy. It leads the acetabuler malplacement in an inadequate coverege. To overcome this problem a method of acetabuloplasty was described (Dunn & Hess, 1976; Hartofilakidis et al., 1988; Stamos et al., 1984). They termed this technique as cotyloplasty. In this technique, they created a controlled comminuted fracture of the entire medial wall of the acetabulum with use of a reamer or a chisel after compilation of the acetabuler reaming. Perforating the internal layer of the periosteum was avoided. After obtaining a large amount of autogenous cancellous graft from femoral head, they placed the graft material over the periosteum of the fractured medial wall. They finally cemented the acetabuler component at an angle of 40-45 degrees horizontally and 10 degrees of anteversion. They adviced 3 to 4 weeks bed rest postoperatively and didn't allow full weight bearing until the graft is incorparated radiographically, considering the horizontal compressive vectors applied by the muscles of the hip. Hartofilakidis et al. used this technique in 68 total hip operation which they used Charnley implants, and Charnley technique, involves an osteotomy of the greater trochanter (Hartofilakidis et al., 1996). Forty nine of the patients were type 3, 31 were type 2 and 6 were type 1 according to their classification. They found good or excellent results in 94 % of the patients operated in a mean duration of follow-up of seven years.

Various types of implants had been attempted in the reconstruction of the acetabulum. Cemented cups were tended to be use in large series in the past. In a series of Stans et al., aseptic loosening developed in 53% of cemented acetabular components (Stans et al., 1998). They thought that this high loosening rates were related with the acetabuler component malplacement in Crowe type III patients. Insertion of the acetabuler component without cement may be preferred when the osseous cavity could provide at least 80 % osseous coverage of a cementless cup (Hartofilakidis & Karachalios, 2004).

Perka et al. used a cementless threaded cups in reconstruction of the acetabulum (Perka et al, 2004). They didn't use a bone graft material to reconstruct the superolateral margin and the cup was slightly medialized to achieve stable anchorage of at least one thread in the existing bone. Although it was found that threaded acetabuler components had high loosing results in the past (Stan et al., 1998), Perka reported a survival rate of % 97.5 at an average of 9.3 years for threaded cups. Their results were better than the those after implantation of cemented cups.

Flecher et al. reported a survival rate of 94.7% at 12 years, using a cementless pres-fit acetabuler component with an obturator hook and screws (Flecher et al., 2008). They sustained that this implant combined the principles of a reinforcement ring with those of uncemented acetabular press-fit components.

2.4.4 The usage of bone grafts in the augmentation of acetabuler component

A technique of bolting the femoral head to the wing of ilium was developed to support the acetabuler component (Harris, 1974). The acetabular cavity was reamed together with into the graft and the host bone. Screws were also used in fixing the autograft. Femoral head allografts became popular in time after the advantages of autografts Jasty & Harris, 1987). It was reported that this technique worked well for short time follow-up and gave the surgeon the possibility of overcoming with the atrophic acetabulums (Harris et al., 1977). However, a high failure rate of nearly 46% were reported at a follow-up of twenty years with the use of the femoral head as an autograft for augmenting the superolateral aspect of the acetabular rim (Harris, 1993; Mulroy & Harris, 1990). The difficulties in revascularisation and of the large grafts and the forces which the graft is exposed may be the possible reasons for the failure. Also, the high failure rates of femoral head augmentation in the reconstruction of superolateral acetabulum with cancellous bone fixation was related with mostly proximal placement of the acetabulum (Stans et al., 1998). Only cement augmentation may be an option in reconstructing the acetabulum in Crowe type III patients. It was reported that cement augmentation works well if the initial hip center is within the true acetabuler region (Stans et al., 1998).

After the cementless acetabuler components began to be used in dysplasia patients, the need to massive grafts in acetabular reconstruction, even at atrophic acetabulums, was diminished (Jasty et al., 1995). It was suggested that lack of osseous reconstruction of the lateral acetabular margin did not have any notable influence on the stability of the cup (Perka et al., 2004). In our personel experiences, if you have press-fit fixation between anterior and posterior wall or sufficient fixation with screws; it is allowed early weight bearing without any problem.

2.4.5 The approach to the deformed femur

The difficulty in reconstructing the femur of dysplastic patients mostly resulted from the alteration in the anatomy of the femur. The femur of the DDH patients were shown to have shorter necks and smaller straighter canals than the normal femurs (Noble et al., 2003). Cemented stems were used in dysplastic patients for a long time with a lesser success than the patients of primer arthrosis. Probably, the biomechanical abnormality of the hip and the persisted limbing after the surgery causes the act of abnormal forces on the cemented component. Consequently early aseptic loosening rates of cemented components increases in DDH patients. In a 20 years follow-up, 5 % aseptic loosing rate was reported with the cemented femoral components (Klapach et al., 2001). Morever evidence of aseptic loosening was observed in 40% of the femoral components of Crowe type III patients at 20 years duration (Stans et al., 1998).

Cementless femoral stems seem to be more useful in reconstruction of young patients. Furthermore usage of the cementless stems prevent the occupation of excessive thick cement in narrow medullary canals. In a series of Lai et al., 56 patients, who have Crowe type 4 DDH, were operated with cementless stems (Lai et al., 2005). They didn't report any stem revision in a follow-up period of mean 12.3 years.

Cementless Zweymüller stem was used in 121 dysplastic hips and fracture occured in the proximal part of the femur in seven cases (Perka et al., 2004). They believed that the high rate of femoral fracture was a result of incresed anteversion of the femoral neck, the tight medullary space and the the altered anatomy in the proximal femur following previous operations. However the survival rate of the stems was not influenced by this complication and it was reported as % 100 at an average follow-up duration of 9.3 years.

The porous coated S-Rom cementless moduler stem was also reported as successful in the treatment of Crowe type III and IV hips, at a 10 year follow-up (Biant et al., 2009). They used the prosthesis as an intramedullary fixation device in the patients whom were required femoral shortening, with the benefit of the straight structure of this stem.

The excessive femoral anteversion seems to be an important problem in DDH patients rather than the primer arthrosis patients (Argenson et al.,2005). Compensating for excessive anteversion of the dysplastic femur is easy with the use of cemented stems. If a cementless stem will be used, it may be better to choose a moduler or distally fixed component rather than proximally fixed femoral component. The proximally fixed components don't allow you to rotate the stem to compansate the anteversion because of the metaphyseal filling.

Moduler stems allow us the regulation of the femoral anteversion unrelated with proximal metaphsial morphology (Cameron et al., 1996). An other option in overcoming the anteversion problem is the usage of the thin conically stems. The results of Wagner conic prosthesis are also found as successful in a short term period (Ström et al, 2003). Hartofilakidis reported successfull results with CDH Charnley prosthesis, a straight thin prosthesis (Hartofilakidis & Karachalios, 2004).

2.4.6 The subtrochanteric femoral shortening osteotomy

The restoration of the acetabulum to the anatomic center of the hip is not always so easy especially in Crowe type 4 patients. Three possible alternative to solve this problem on the dislocated femur were reported; 1) Trochanteric osteotomy may be carried out with metaphysel shortening and advancement of the trochanter. Cemented stem may be the choice of use in this option, 2) A modular stem may be an option, 3) Subtrochanteric shortening and derotation, combined with an distally fixed cementless stem is the third alternative (Cabenala, 2001). Trial reduction by skeletal or skin traction was performed before the surgery, to assess the potential reduction (Symenoides et al., 1997). They also used a gradual traction technique with the use of an external fixator but pain and nerve palsy was reported in this case. According to us, subtrochanteric femoral shortening osteotomy is the best option to lower the femoral head to its original site instead of soft tissue release without damaging the nerves by streching. Non-union rates are low with the use of cementless femoral stems, especially in Crowe type 4 dysplasies. Its also useful in aligning the anteversion of the neck in such malrotated femoral metaphysises. There is more than one technique reported for the shortening of the femur (Bruce et al., 2000; Klisic & Jankovic, 1976; Sener et al., 2002; Yasgur et al.,1997). Klisic and Jankovic (Klisic & Jankovic, 1976) was first stated the usage of the femoral shortening osteotomies in the treatment of highly dislocated hips and than it was adapted into the total hip replacement operations by Sponseller and MacBeath (Sponseller & McBeath, 1988). Transvers subtrochanteric shortening osteotomy is a successful technique and none neurologic complication was reported in a series of Myung- Sik Park et al. of 24 patients operated with transvers osteotomy (Park et al., 2007). Yalcin et al. reported 79,5 % good and perfect results in 44 total hip replacements accompanied by transvers osteotomy at a meanly 62 months follow-up (Yalcin et al., 2010). In a study of Aeron et al., the patients, whom femurs were shortened, were followed up to mean 4.8 years and preoperative Harris scores found to increase from 43 to 89, postoperatively (Krych et al., 2010).

The short time requirement for bone healing, much bone contact and stability against the torsional forces are the advantages of step-cut osteotomy. Despite of these advantages, Sener et al. reported 2 non-unions after step-cut osteotomy in 28 patients (Sener et al., 2002) while one non-union was reported after transvers osteotomy in 14 hips (Onodera et al., 2006). In an other serie, Masaki Takao et al. combined cementless moduler total hip prosthesis with step-cut subtrochanteric shortening osteotomy (Takao et al., 2011). No non-union and nerve palsy were reported. Merle d'Aubigne and Postel hip score increased from 9 to 16 in this 23 cases serie. The operation found to be successfull in Crowe type IV patients. Furthermore, Grappiolo et al performed different femoral osteotomy techniques during total hip prosthesis surgery of 128 dysplastic hips (Grappiolo et al, 2007). They thought that subtrochanteric transvers osteotomy was the safest technique, after a 20 years experience.

Also, subtrochanteric transvers osteotomy is the technique which was favoured in our clinic for last 6 and 7 years. It seems to be much easy to perform, rather than the other techniques. The other advantage of this technique is that it gives you the possibility to fix the malrotation of the proximally femur.

In spite of these good results with shortening osteotomy, some authors don't favor shorthening of the femoral diaphysis (Hartofilakidis & Karachalios, 2004). Osteotomy of the greater trochanter was performed in all hips except for three with dysplasia in a series of Hartofilakidis, consisted of 223 patients. They shortened the femur with progressive resection of bone from the femoral neck. Although they acquired a limb-lengthening of average 3.5 cm (1 to 7 cm) in the high dislocated patients, they only reported 2 nerve palsy which resolved within six months. They believed that nerve damage can be avoided by cautious handling of the retractors intraoperatively and by the placement of both hip and knee in flexion for three to four days after the operation. Fibrous union was seen 4%, 13% and 22% of the patients in dysplastic, low dislocated and high dislocated groups, respectively. It was stated that all of these fibrous unions were asymptomatic. Non-union and migration of the greater trochanter was observed in 2 and 1 hips in low dislocated and high dislocated groups, respectively.

Kerboull et al., also performed femoral stem mostly without shortening in 118 Crowe type IV hips (Kerboull et al., 2001). Shortening of the femur was needed only in 2 patients. Only 1 transient peroneal nevre palsy was reported although limb was lengthened more than 4 cm in 30 hips. The amount of limb lengthening causing nerve palsy, is not clear in the literature. After the operation, hip and knee flexion may help in reducing the tension in femoral and peroneal nerve, respectively. It was reported that 2.7 cm lengthening increased the risk of peroneal nerve injury, while 4.4 cm lengthening increased the risk of sciatic nerve injury (Edwards et al., 1987). They concluded that the maximal lengthening shouldn't exceed 4 cm. The 30 % of nerve palsy thought to be due to lengthening of the limb (Johanson et al., 1983). However, no correlation was observed between nerve injury and the amount of limb lengthening in a study, recently (Eggli et al, 1999). They found out the relation between nerve injury and the severity of the surgery. All cases who had nerve palsy after the operation, except one, required hard work because of different reasons like; previous operation, the severity of the disease, large acetabuler defect, serious flexion deformity of the hip. Direct or indirect mechanical trauma was thougth to be responsible in nerve palsy.

2.4.7 The resurfacing arthroplasty in DDH

Although that total hip arthroplasty is known as the golden treatment option in DDH, it was reported that resurfacing arthroplasty would be a successful alternative in Crowe type 1-2 patients (Xu et al., 2008). Amsutz et al. operated 103 hips of 90 patients whom have 94 percent Crowe type 1 displasia and reported it as a perfect method in a short and mid term period (Amstutz et al., 2008). It was interesting that the 43% of the femoral heads had a defect of more than 1 cm in their series. The vitality of the femoral head of the patients, whom were operated with Birmingham implants, was examined by fluride positron emission tomography and found that the femoral head vitality persisted after the operation (Forrest et al., 2006). However, the ALVAL reaction resulted from metal-metal implants is the drawback of this technique, because the age-group of the indicated patients are mostly young.

2.4.8 Difficulties of arthroplasty in previously operated patients

The affect of the previous operations at the childhood on arthroplasty is not clear. Highly complication and revision rates were reported after total hip arthroplasty of the patients with femoral osteotomy (Ferguson et al., 1994). Boos et al. compared the results of the total hip arthroplasty between the patients whom femoral osteomy was performed before and not performed (Boos et al., 1997). There was no difference in peri-operatif complication and revision rates but they stated that the operation time was much longer and the surgical exposure was much difficult in the previously operated group than the other.

Chiari osteotomy was thought to be as an ease in the acetabuler component placement during the arthroplasty operations (Chiari, 1974). Supporters of this opinion attract the attention on the need of long time studies to sustain their theory (Hoffman et al., 1974; Mitchell, 1974; Wedge, 1995). Despite of these supporters, more bleeding was reported in previously operated patients with Chiari technique. And it was also stated that it was time consuming and the morbidiy was higher (Minoda et al., 2006). The removal of the implants used during the osteotomy operations seems as a factor increasing the morbidity (Beaupre & Csongradi, 1996; Jago & Hindley, 1998). In our experience, it is hard to secure the primary stability of the acetabulum in patients who had periacetabular osteotomy beforehand.

3. Conclusion

There are several classification systems which may tell us the pathology very well in DDH. However none of them seems to be a candidate to guide for the surgeon in choosing the best technique and prosthesis as well. It is obvious that there is a need for a new classification method in DDH. 3D CT scans may be useful in preoperative planning. The reconstruction in DDH will remain as a challange which may be overcomed in the battle field since a new classification method is reported to help the surgeon.

4. References

Anda S., Terjesen T., Kvistad K.A. (1991). Computed tomography measurements of the acetabulum in adult dysplastic hips: which level is appropriate? *Skeletal Radiol.* Vol.20, No.4, pp.267-271, ISBN 1853218

Amstutz HC, Le Duff MJ, Harvey N, Hoberg M. (2008). Improved survivorship of hybrid metal-on-metal hip resurfacing with second-generation techniques for Crowe-I and II developmental dysplasia of the hip. *J Bone Joint Surg Am.* Vol.90, Suppl. 3, (August), pp.12-20, ISBN 18676931

Argenson JN, Ryembault E, Flecher X, Brassart N, Parratte S, Aubaniac JM. (2005). Three-dimensional anatomy of the hip in osteoarthritis after developmental dysplasia. *J Bone Joint Surg Br.* Vol.87, No.9, (September), pp.1192-1196, ISBN 16129740

Beaupre G.S., Csongradi J.J. (1996). Refracture risk after plate removal in the forearm. *J Orthop Trauma.* Vol.10, No.2, (February), pp.87-92, ISBN 8932666

Biant L.C., Bruce W.J., Assini J.B., Walker P.M., Walsh W.R. (2009). Primary total hip arthroplasty in severe developmental dysplasia of the hip. Ten-year results using a cementless modular stem. *J Arthroplasty.* Vol.24, No.1, (January), pp.27-32, ISBN 18977633

Boos N., Krushell R., Ganz R., Müller M.E. (1997). Total hip arthroplasty after previous proximal femoral osteotomy. *J Bone Joint Surg Br*. Vol.79, No.2, (March), pp.247-253, ISBN 9119851

Bozic K.J., Freiberg A.A., Harris W.H. (2004).The high hip center. *Clin Orthop Relat Res*. Vol.420, (March), pp.101-105, ISBN 15057084

Bruce W.J., Rizkallah S.M., Kwon Y.M., Goldberg J.A., Walsh W.R. (2000). A new technique of subtrochanteric shortening in total hip arthroplasty: surgical technique and results of 9 cases. *J Arthroplasty*. Vol.15, No.5, (August), pp.617-626, ISBN 10960001

Brunner A, Ulmar B, Reichel H, Decking R. (2008). The Eftekhar and Kerboul classifications in assessment of developmental dysplasia of the hip in adult patients. Measurement of inter- and intraobserver reliability. *HSS J*. Vol.4, No.1, (February), pp.25-31, ISBN 18751859

Cabanela M.E. (2001) Total hip arthroplasty for developmental dysplasia of the hip. *Orthopedics*. Vol.24, No.9, (September) pp.865-866, ISBN 11570460

Charnley J., Feagin J.A. (1973). Low-friction arthroplasty in congenital subluxation of the hip. *Clin Orthop Relat Res*. Vol.91, (March-April), pp.98-113, ISBN 4574070

Cameron H.U., Botsford D.J., Park Y.S. (1996). Influence of the Crowe rating on the outcome of total hip arthroplasty in congenital hip dysplasia. *J Arthroplasty*. Vol.11, No.5, (August), pp.582-587, ISBN 8872579

Chougle A., Hemmady M.V., Hodgkinson J.P. (2005). Severity of hip dysplasia and loosening of the socket in cemented total hip replacement. A long-term follow-up. *J Bone Joint Surg Br*. Vol.87, No.1, (January), pp.16-20, ISBN 15686231

Chiari K. (1974). Medial displacement osteotomy of the pelvis. *Clin Orthop Relat Res*. Vol.98, (January-Febuary), pp.55-71, ISBN 4817245

Crowe J.F., Mani V.J., Ranawat C.S. (1979). Total hip replacement in congenital dislocation and dysplasia of the hip. *J Bone Joint Surg Am*. Vol.61, No.1, (January), pp.15-23, ISBN 365863

Dearborn J.T., Harris W.H. (1999). High placement of an acetabular component inserted without cement in a revision total hip arthroplasty. Results after a mean of ten years. *J Bone Joint Surg Am*. Apr;81(4):469-80, ISBN 10225792

Decking R, Brunner A, Decking J, Puhl W, Günther KP. (2006). Reliability of the Crowe und Hartofilakidis classifications used in the assessment of the adult dysplastic hip. *Skeletal Radiol*. Vol.35, No.5, (May), pp.282-287, ISBN 16534641

Doehring T.C., Rubash H.E., Shelley F.J., Schwendeman L.J., Donaldson T.K., Navalgund Y.A. (1996). Effect of superior and superolateral relocations of the hip center on hip joint forces. An experimental and analytical analysis. *J Arthroplasty*. Vol.11, No.6, (September), pp.693-703, ISBN 8884445

Dudkiewicz I., Salai M., Ganel A., Blankstein A., Chechik A. (2002). Total hip arthroplasty in patients younger than 30 years of age following developmental dysplasia of hip (DDH) in infancy. *Arch Orthop Trauma Surg*. Vol.122, No.3, (April), pp.139-142, ISBN 11927994

Dunn HK, Hess WE. (1976). Total hip reconstruction in chronically dislocated hips. *J Bone Joint Surg Am*. Vol.58, No.6, (September), pp.838-845, ISBN 956229

Edwards BN, Tullos HS, Noble PC. (1987). Contributory factors and etiology of sciatic nerve palsy in total hip arthroplasty. *Clin Orthop Relat Res.* Vol.218, (May), pp.136-141, ISBN 3568473

Eftekhar N. (1978). Principles of total hip arthroplasty. C V Mosby, St. Louis, pp 437–455.

Eggli S., Hankemayer S., Müller M.E. (1999). Nerve palsy after leg lengthening in total replacement arthroplasty for developmental dysplasia of the hip. *J Bone Joint Surg Br.* Vol.81, No.5, (September), pp.843-845, ISBN 10530847

Ferguson G.M., Cabanela M.E., Ilstrup D.M. (1994). Total hip arthroplasty after failed intertrochanteric osteotomy. *J Bone Joint Surg Br.* Vol.76, No.2, pp.252-257, ISBN 8113286

Flecher X., Parratte S., Brassart N., Aubaniac J.M., Argenson J.N. (2008). Evaluation of the hip center in total hip arthroplasty for old developmental dysplasia. *J Arthroplasty.* Vol.23, No.8, (December), pp.1189-1196, ISBN 18534475

Forrest N., Welch A., Murray AD., Schweiger L., Hutchison J., Ashcroft G.P. (2006). Femoral head viability after Birmingham resurfacing hip arthroplasty: assessment with use of [18F] fluoride positron emission tomography. *J Bone Joint Surg Am.* Vol.88, Suppl.3, (November), pp.84-89, ISBN 17079372

Gardner E., Gray D.J. (1950). Prenatal development of the human hip joint. *Am J Anat.* Vol.87, No.2, (September), pp.163-211, ISBN 14771010

Gill T.J., Sledge J.B., Müller M.E. (1998). Total hip arthroplasty with use of an acetabular reinforcement ring in patients who have congenital dysplasia of the hip. Results at five to fifteen years. *J Bone Joint Surg Am.* Vol.80, No.7, (July), pp.969-979, ISBN 9698001

Grappiolo G., Spotorno L., Burastero G. (2007). Evolution of surgical techniques for the treatment of angular and torsional deviation in DDH: 20 years experience. *Hip Int.* Vol.17, Suppl.5, pp.105-110, ISBN 19197890

Harris W.H. (1974). Total hip replacement for congenital dysplasia of the hip: Technique. *In* W.H. Harris (Ed). *The Hip, Proceedings of the 2nd Open Scientific Session of the Hip Society.* St Louis, CV Mosby, pp.251-265

Harris W.H., Crothers O., Oh I. (1977). Total hip replacement and femoral-head bone-grafting for severe acetabular deficiency in adults. *J Bone Joint Surg Am.* Vol.59, No.6, (September), pp.752-759, ISBN 908698

Harris W.H. (1993). Management of the deficient acetabulum using cementless fixation without bone grafting. *Orthop Clin North Am.* Vol.24, No.4, (October), pp.663-665, ISBN 8414432

Harrison T.J. (1961). The influence of the femoral head on pelvic growth and acetabular form in the rat. *J Anat.* Vol.95, (January), pp.12-24, ISBN 13711848

Hartofilakidis G., Stamos K, Ioannidis T.T. (1988). Low friction arthroplasty for old untreated congenital dislocation of the hip. *J Bone Joint Surg Br.* Vol.70, No.2, (March), pp.182-186, ISBN 3346284

Hartofilakidis G., Stamos K., Karachalios T., Ioannidis T.T., Zacharakis N. (1996). Congenital hip disease in adults. Classification of acetabular deficiencies and operative treatment with acetabuloplasty combined with total hip arthroplasty. *J Bone Joint Surg Am.* Vol.78, No.5, (May), pp.683-92, ISBN 8642024

Hartofilakidis G., Karachalios T., Stamos K.G. (2000). Epidemiology, demographics, and natural history of congenital hip disease in adults. *Orthopedics.* Vol.23, No.8, (August), pp.823-7, ISBN 10952045

Hartofilakidis G., Karachalios T. (2004). Total hip arthroplasty for congenital hip disease. *J Bone Joint Surg Am.* Vol.86-A, No.2, (February), pp.242-250, ISBN 14960667

Hess W.E., Umber J.S. (1978). Total hip arthroplasty in chronically dislocated hips. Follow-up study on the protrusio socket technique. *J Bone Joint Surg Am.* Vol.60, No.7, (October), pp.948-954, ISBN 701343

Heyman C.H., Herndon C.H. (1950). Legg-Perthes disease; a method for the measurement of the roentgenographic result. *J Bone Joint Surg Am.* Vol.32, No.A4, (October), pp.767-778, ISBN 14784485

Hirakawa K., Mitsugi N., Koshino T., Saito T., Hirasawa Y., Kubo T. (2001). Effect of acetabular cup position and orientation in cemented total hip arthroplasty. *Clin Orthop Relat Res.* Vol.388, (July), pp.135-142, ISBN 11451112

Hoffman D.V., Simmons E.H., Barrington T.W. (1974). The results of the Chiari osteotomy. *Clin Orthop Relat Res.* Vol.98, (January-February), pp.162-170, ISBN 4817226

Jago E.R., Hindley C.J. (1998). The removal of metalwork in children. *Injury.* Vol.29, No.6, (July), pp.439-441, ISBN 9813700

Jasty M., Harris W.H. (1990). Salvage total hip reconstruction in patients with major acetabular bone deficiency using structural femoral head allografts. J Bone Joint Surg Br. Vol.72, No.1, (January), pp.63-67, ISBN 2298796

Jasty M., Anderson M.J., Harris W.H. (1995). Total hip replacement for developmental dysplasia of the hip. Clin Orthop Relat Res. Vol.311, (February), pp.40-45, ISBN 7634589

Johanson N.A., Pellicci P.M., Tsairis P., Salvati E.A. (1983). Nerve injury in total hip arthroplasty. *Clin Orthop Relat Res.* Vol.179, (October), pp.214-222, ISBN 6617020

Kennedy J.G., Rogers W.B., Soffe K.E., Sullivan R.J., Griffen D.G., Sheehan L.J. (1998). Effect of acetabular component orientation on recurrent dislocation, pelvic osteolysis, polyethylene wear, and component migration. *J Arthroplasty.* Vol.13, No.5, (August), pp.530-534, ISBN 9726318

Kerboul M., Mathieu M., Sauzieres P. (1987). Total hip replacement for congenital dislocation of the hip. In: Postel M., Kerboul M., Evrard J., Courpied J.P. (eds) Total hip replacement. Springer, Berlin Heidelberg New York, pp 51–66 .

Kerboull M., Hamadouche M., Kerboull L. (2001). Total hip arthroplasty for Crowe type IV developmental hip dysplasia: a long-term follow-up study. *J Arthroplasty.* Vol.16, No.8, Suppl. 1, (December), pp.170-176, ISBN 11742471

Klapach A.S., Callaghan J.J., Goetz D.D., Olejniczak J.P., Johnston R.C.(2001). Charnley total hip arthroplasty with use of improved cementing techniques: a minimum twenty-year follow-up study. *J Bone Joint Surg Am.* Vol.83-A, No.12, (December), pp.1840-1848, ISBN 11741064

Klisic P., Jankovic L. (1976). Combined procedure of open reduction and shortening of the femur in treatment of congenital dislocation of the hips in older children. *Clin Orthop Relat Res.* Vol.119, (September), pp.60-69, ISBN 954325

Krych A.J., Howard J.L., Trousdale R.T., Cabanela M.E., Berry D.J. (2010). Total hip arthroplasty with shortening subtrochanteric osteotomy in Crowe type-IV developmental dysplasia: surgical technique. *J Bone Joint Surg Am.* Suppl. 1, Pt. 2, (September), pp.176-187, ISBN 20844173

Kumar A., Shair A.B. (1997). An extended iliofemoral approach for total arthroplasty in late congenital dislocation of the hip: a case report. *Int Orthop.* Vol.21, No.4, (September), pp.265-266, ISBN 9349966

Lai K.A., Shen W.J., Huang L.W., Chen M.Y. (2005). Cementless total hip arthroplasty and limb-length equalization in patients with unilateral Crowe type-IV hip dislocation. *J Bone Joint Surg Am.* Vol.87, No.2, (February), pp.339-345, ISBN 15687157

Linde F., Jensen J. (1988). Socket loosening in arthroplasty for congenital dislocation of the hip. *Acta Orthop Scand.* Vol.59, No.3, (June), pp.254-257, ISBN 3381653

MacKenzie J.R., Kelley S.S., Johnston R.C. (1996). Total hip replacement for coxarthrosis secondary to congenital dysplasia and dislocation of the hip. Long-term results. *J Bone Joint Surg Am.* Vol.78, No.1, (January), pp.55-61, ISBN 8550680

McQueary F.G., Johnston R.C. (1988). Coxarthrosis after congenital dysplasia. Treatment by total hip arthroplasty without acetabular bone-grafting. *J Bone Joint Surg Am.* Vol.70, No.8, (September), pp.1140-1144, ISBN 3417699

Mendes D.G., Said M.S., Aslan K. (1996). Classification of adult congenital hip dysplasia for total hip arthroplasty. *Orthopedics.* Vol.19, No.10, (October), pp. 881-887, ISBN 8905863

Minoda Y., Kadowaki T., Kim M. (2006). Total hip arthroplasty of dysplastic hip after previous Chiari pelvic osteotomy. *Arch Orthop Trauma Surg.* Vol.126, No.6, (August), pp.394-400, ISBN 16628429

Mitchell G.P. (1974). Chiari medial displacement osteotomy. *Clin Orthop Relat Res.* Vol.98, (January-February), pp.146-150, ISBN 4817224

Mulroy R.D. Jr., Harris W.H. (1990). Failure of acetabular autogenous grafts in total hip arthroplasty. Increasing incidence: a follow-up note. *J Bone Joint Surg Am.* Vol.72, No.10, (December), pp.1536-1540, ISBN 2254363

Nakamura S., Yorikawa J., Otsuka K., Takeshita K., Harasawa A., Matsushita T. (2000). Evaluation of acetabular dysplasia using a top view of the hip on three-dimensional CT. *J Orthop Sci.* Vol.5, No.6, (November), pp.533-539, ISBN 11180914

Noble P.C., Kamaric E., Sugano N., Matsubara M., Harada Y., Ohzono K., Paravic V. (2003). Three-dimensional shape of the dysplastic femur: implications for THR. *Clin Orthop Relat Res.* Vol.417, (December), pp.27-40,ISBN 14646700

Onodera S., Majima T., Ito H., Matsuno T., Kishimoto T., Minami A. (2006). Cementless total hip arthroplasty using the modular S-ROM prosthesis combined with corrective proximal femoral osteotomy. *J Arthroplasty.* Vol.21, No.5, (August), pp.664-669, ISBN 16877151

Paavilainen T., Hoikka V., Solonen K.A. (1990). Cementless total replacement for severely dysplastic or dislocated hips. *J Bone Joint Surg Br*. Vol.72, No.2, (March), pp.205-211, ISBN 2312556

Pagnano W., Hanssen A.D., Lewallen D.G., Shaughnessy W.J. (1996). The effect of superior placement of the acetabular component on the rate of loosening after total hip arthroplasty. *J Bone Joint Surg Am*. Vol.78, No.7, (July), pp.1004-14, ISBN 8698717

Park M.S., Kim K.H., Jeong W.C. (2007). Transverse subtrochanteric shortening osteotomy in primary total hip arthroplasty for patients with severe hip developmental dysplasia. *J Arthroplasty*. Vol.22, No.7, (October), pp.1031-1036, ISBN 17920477

Patterson F.P., Brown C.S. (1972). The McKee-Farrar total hip replacement. Preliminary results and complications of 368 operations performed in five general hospitals. *J Bone Joint Surg Am*. Vol.54, No.2, (March), pp.257-75, ISBN 4631242

Perka C., Fischer U., Taylor W.R., Matziolis G. (2004). Developmental hip dysplasia treated with total hip arthroplasty with a straight stem and a threaded cup. *J Bone Joint Surg Am*. Vol.86-A, No.2, (February), pp.312-319, ISBN 14960676

Ponseti I.V. (1978). Growth and development of the acetabulum in the normal child. Anatomical, histological, and roentgenographic studies. *J Bone Joint Surg Am*. Vol.60, No.5, (July), pp.575-585. ISBN 681376

Rális Z., McKibbin B. (1973). Changes in shape of the human hip joint during its development and their relation to its stability. *J Bone Joint Surg Br*. Vol.55, No.4, (November), pp.780-785, ISBN 4766182

Russotti G.M., Harris W.H. (1991). Proximal placement of the acetabular component in total hip arthroplasty. A long-term follow-up study. *J Bone Joint Surg Am*. Vol.73, No.4, (April), pp. 587-592, ISBN 2013598

Sharp I. (1961). Acetabular dysplasia. *J Bone Joint Surg (Br)*. Vol.43, pp.268-272.

Saikko V.O. (1995). Wear of the polyethylene acetabular cup. The effect of head material, head diameter, and cup thickness studied with a hip simulator. *Acta Orthop Scand*. Vol.66, No.6, (December), pp.501-506, ISBN 8553815

Sener N., Tozun I.R., Asik M. (2002). Femoral shortening and cementless arthroplasty in high congenital dislocation of the hip. *J Arthroplasty*. Vol.17, No.1, (January), pp.41-48, ISBN 11805923

Smith W.S., Ireton R.J, Coleman C.R. (1958). Sequelae of experimental dislocation of a weight-bearing ball- and socket joint in a young growing animal; gross alterations in bone and cartilage. *J Bone Joint Surg Am*. Vol.40-A, No.5, (October), pp.1121-1127, ISBN 13587581

Sponseller P.D., McBeath A.A. (1988). Subtrochanteric osteotomy with intramedullary fixation for arthroplasty of the dysplastic hip. A case report. *J Arthroplasty*. Vol.3, No.4, pp.351-354, ISBN 3241173

Stamos K., Hartofilakidis G., Koroneas A., Xenakis T. Mechanical strength of P.M.M.A bonding to cancellous bone graft. An experimental study in dogs. Read the combined meetings of the Hellenic Association of Orthopaedic Surgery and Traumatology and American Hip Society, Rhodes, May 4, 1984.

Stans A.A., Pagnano M.W., Shaughnessy W.J., Hanssen A.D. (1998). Results of total hip arthroplasty for Crowe Type III developmental hip dysplasia. *Clin Orthop Relat Res.* Vol.348, (March), pp.149-157, ISBN 9553547

Strayer L.M. (1943). The Embryology of the Human Hip Joint. *Yale J Biol Med.* Vol.16, No.1, (October 1943), pp. 13-26.6, ISBN 21434122

Ström H., Mallmin H., Milbrink J., Petrén-Mallmin M., Nivbrant B., Kolstad K. (2003). The cone hip stem: a prospective study of 13 patients followed for 5 years with RSA. Acta Orthop Scand. Vol.74, No.5, (October), pp.525-530, ISBN 14620971

Symeonides P.P., Pournaras J., Petsatodes G., Christoforides J., Hatzokos I., Pantazis E. (1997). Total hip arthroplasty in neglected congenital dislocation of the hip. *Clin Orthop Relat Res.* Vol.341, (August), pp.55-61, ISBN 9269155

Takao M., Ohzono K., Nishii T., Miki H., Nakamura N., Sugano N. (2011). Cementless modular total hip arthroplasty with subtrochanteric shortening osteotomy for hips with developmental dysplasia. *J Bone Joint Surg Am.* Vol.93, No.6, (March), pp.548-555, ISBN 21411705

Troelsen A, Rømer L, Jacobsen S, Ladelund S, Søballe K. (2010). Cranial acetabular retroversion is common in developmental dysplasia of the hip as assessed by the weight bearing position. *Acta Orthop.* Vol.81, No.4, (August), pp.436-441, ISBN 20809742

Watanabe RS. (1974). Embryology of the Human Hip. *Clin Orthop Relat Res.* Vol.98, (Jan-Feb), pp.8-26, ISBN 4817247

Wedge J.H. (1995). Osteotomy of the pelvis for the management of hip disease in young adults. *Can J Surg.* Vol.38, Suppl.1, (February), pp.25-32, ISBN 7874625

Wedge J.H., Wasylenko M.J. (1978). The natural history of congenital dislocation of the hip: a critical review. *Clin Orthop Relat Res.* Vol.137, (Nov-Dec), pp.154-162, ISBN 743823

Weinstein S.L. (1987). Natural history of congenital hip dislocation (CDH) and hip dysplasia. *Clin Orthop Relat Res.* Vol.225, (December), pp.62-76. ISBN 3315382

Wiberg G. (1939). Studies on dysplasiic acelabula and congenital subluxation of the hip joint. *Acta Ortbop Scand.* Vol. 58, No. Suppl, pp.1-132

Xenakis TA, Gelalis ID, Koukoubis TD, Soucacos PN, Vartziotis K, Kontoyiannis D, Tatsis C. (1996). Neglected congenital dislocation of the hip. Role of computed tomography and computer-aided design for total hip arthroplasty. *J Arthroplasty.* Vol.11, No.8, (December), pp.893-8, ISBN 8986566

Xu W.D., Li J., Zhou Z.H., Wu Y.S., Li M. (2008). Results of hip resurfacing for developmental dysplasia of the hip of Crowe type I and II. *Chin Med J (Engl).* Vol.121, No.15, (August), pp.1379-1383, ISBN 18959113

Yalcin N., Kilicarslan K., Karatas F., Mutlu T., Yildirim H. (2010). Cementless total hip arthroplasty with subtrochanteric transverse shortening osteotomy for severely dysplastic or dislocated hips. *Hip Int.* Vol.20, No.1, (January-March), pp.87-93, ISBN 20235079

Yasgur D.J., Stuchin S.A., Adler E.M., DiCesare P.E. (1997). Subtrochanteric femoral shortening osteotomy in total hip arthroplasty for high-riding developmental dislocation of the hip. *J Arthroplasty.* Vol.12, No.8, (December), pp.880-888, ISBN 9458253

Yoder S.A., Brand R.A., Pedersen D.R., O'Gorman T.W. (1988). Total hip acetabular component position affects component loosening rates. *Clin Orthop Relat Res.* Vol.228, (March), pp.79-87, ISBN 3342591

11

Hip Arthroplasty in Highly Dislocated Hips

Zoran Bascarevic[1,2], Zoran Vukasinovic[1,2],
Violeta Bascarevic[2] and Vladimir Bascarevic[1,3]
[1]Faculty of Medicine, University of Belgrade, Belgrade
[2]Institute of Orthopaedic Surgery „Banjica", Belgrade
[3]Institute of Neurosurgery, Clinical Center of Serbia, Belgrade
Serbia

1. Introduction

Developmental disorder of the hip (DDH) is the most frequent disease of this joint. It is manifested by dysplasia, subluxation or luxation in childhood period and arthrosis in adults. Early degenerative changes of the hip occur at the location of disordered anatomy and biomechanics already in youth, while in the childhood age they are mostly asymptomatic (Ando & Gotoh, 1990).

DDH mostly occurs in females, even 4-10 times more often than in males. Also, the disease is unevenly expanded, both ethnically and geographically, but also according to different habits in regard to the nursing care of neonates and infants. For example, the disease does not develop among the Bantu colored population, while in Canadian Indians it is very frequent rating even 12.3%, which is related to their habit of nursing babies in narrow wooden cradles. In those Indians who do not practice it the frequency is considerably lower (1.2%) (Vukasinovic et al., 1994, 2004).

In our regions data on the frequency of DDH vary between 0.5-34.8%, depending on the regional customs in nursing children, but also on the method applied in the diagnostics of the disease; clinically it is the lowest, radiographically higher, and ultrasonographically the highest (Klisic et al., 1984). Former classical term of the disease was "congenital dislocation of the hip", which, over the years became unsustainable, since it has been disclosed that the disease is not congenital, but that it often develops after birth under the influence of environmental factors. In addition, it does not always involve a total dislocation, but only disturbed interrelationship among the joint surfaces of the hip. Although the former term can be still found in the literature, today the term "developmental disorder of the hip" is accepted worldwide (Klisic, 1989).

2. Etiopathogenesis and pathoanatomy of DDH

To understand the problem faced by the arthroplastic surgeon in treating a high luxation of the hip in adults, it is necessary to be acquainted with etiopathogenesis of the disease, because it is in a direct association with its pathoanatomic substrate.

After numerous years of research, attitudes of the leading world experts on this disease have been mostly brought in accordance (Ando & Gotoh 1990; Cherney & Westin 1989; Klisic et al. 1984, 1989; Vukasinovic & Bascarevic, 2004).

There is the predominating opinion that two groups of etiological factors contribute to the development of DDH; endogenous and exogenous (mechanical). (Vukasinovic & Djoric, 1994; Vukasinovic & Bascarevic, 2004).

Endogenous factors involve acetabular dysplasia, increased anteversion of the femoral neck and head, as well as joint laxity. Beside primary acetabular dysplasia, which is one of the causes of the disease, the so called secondary acetabular dysplasia is also mentioned, which develops due to hip dislocation itself. Although a lax joint capsule can be generalized, as for example when associated with Ehlers-Danlos syndrome, in DDH it is mostly only elongated in the superior-posterior portion, thus secondary, caused by luxation instead of being its major cause. (Vukasinovic & Djoric, 1994; Vukasinovic & Bascarevic, 2004).

Exogenous (mechanical) factors involve the basis of the so called mechanical theory which has been obtaining a rising number of supporters as it can explain the frequency of luxations in first pregnancies, pelvic positions, Cesarean section, high birth weight, oligohydramnion and fetopelvic disproportion. In addition, hip luxation due to DDH is often associated with other deformities of the feet, knees, neck (torticollis) and other. (Vukasinovic & Djoric, 1994; Vukasinovic & Bascarevic, 2004).

Exogenous (mechanical) factors can affect the fetus intrauterine, during delivery and postnatally. The intrauterine factors mostly involve three luxating fetal positions, while the postnatal ones above all refer to traditional baby diapering with bent knees and extended legs. Not only can such a position induce a spontaneous reduction of unstable joint, but it can also provoke the development of luxation. The mechanical factors occurring during birth can be discarded today, because even in newborns the hips are so stable that rough manual manipulation will sooner cause femoral head epyphysiolisis or diaphyseal fracture than hip luxation. It is considered that action of two factors is necessary for DDH to develop; a specific position of the femur involving the head which is not orientated toward the base of the acetabulum and expulsion force pushing the baby's head out of the acetabulum. (Vukasinovic & Djoric, 1994; Vukasinovic & Bascarevic, 2004).

In short, DDH pathogenesis features the following: a predisposing base representing unstable genetic factors, above all acetabular dysplasia and capsular laxity, while the determinant mechanical factors exert pressure on the great trochanter in one of the luxating fetal positions. This can explain the growing incidence of bilateral luxations in pelvic births; forces act on both great trochanters, i.e. isolated left-sided luxations in normal birth (baby head down presentation with left turned back); the maternal promontorium exerting pressure on the great trochanter. (Vukasinovic & Djoric, 1994; Vukasinovic & Bascarevic, 2004).

Pathological changes involve all structures of the joint, while the pathoanatomical substrate differs depending on the degree of disorder.

The acetabulum changes in depth during physiological development becoming the shallowest in the perinatal period. Spherical formation (joint congruency) is caused by the presence and pressure of the femoral head. In DDH unfavorable intra-articular relationships lead to acetabular anterior and superior deficiency, as well as its anteversion. Consequently, the acetabulum becomes ovoid or even triangle-like insufficiently covering the femoral head. It is mostly dilated, but can be also completely undeveloped, narrowed due to the lack of developmental stimulation caused by the absent head in the joint. (Vukasinovic & Djoric, 1994; Bascarevic & Vukasinovic, 2004).

The limbus gradually flattens and thickens first in the superoposterior portion. Gradually, a groove is formed enabling the head to slide out of the joint. It is partially grown together with the capsule and is lacking in some areas. In subluxations it is everted, while in full luxations it is inverted and interpolated between the head and the acetabulum. (Vukasinovic & Djoric, 1994; Bascarevic & Vukasinovic, 2004).

The ligamentum teres differs depending on the severity of disorder ranging from normal and occasionally hypoplastic, elongated and hypertrophic, up to fully atrophic in luxations.

The femoral head can be differently formed, from normal - spherical to flattened and deformed with limbal impression. It is most often decreased with highly expressed fovea. (Vukasinovic & Djoric, 1994; Bascarevic & Vukasinovic, 2004).

The femoral neck is usually shortened with increased anteversion. However, it can even be normal, but also retroverted. The collo-diaphyseal angle is usually normal, but can be also decreased or conversely increased.

The capsule of the joint is thickened and mostly lax, but can be also tightened. With the progression of luxation, it becomes lengthened and narrowed in the empty space between the head and the acetabulum resuming the form of a sand-clock. It grows adhering to the bones that form the acetabulum, thus impeding reduction. (Vukasinovic & Djoric, 1994; Bascarevic & Vukasinovic, 2004).

The ligamentum transversum is most frequently strong and thickened and additionally narrows the already dysplastic acetabulum. Its position is the only constant one in the pathological anatomy of the hip in high luxations and represents the major and occasionally the only orientation point in the attempt to find the true acetabulum in the total arthroplasty of the hip. (Bascarevic & Vukasinovic, 2004).

Muscular motion starters are also changed, particularly the iliopsoas; its tendon is short and thickened, while short external rotators are hypotrophic, but also shortened. However, the major hip abductors, primarily the gluteus medius, although hypotrophic, are not shortened and do not create resistance before reduction. In addition, after arthroplasty and induction of the necessary muscular length (close to physiological) they show unusual vitality in the restitution of strength and function of joints. (Vukasinovic & Djoric, 1994; Bascarevic & Vukasinovic, 2004).

Finally, when we speak of high luxations of the hip in the light of aloarthroplasty, attention should be turned to the fact that DDH is not the only condition causing high luxation of the hip in adults. Hip trauma, juvenile rheumatism, neonatal sepsis and some other similar conditions can also cause established hip luxation that can be resolved only when treated by a total hip arthroplasty (Besset et al., 2003; Betz et al., 1990; Choi et al., 1990; Learmonth et al., 1989; Maric & Haynes 1993; Ruddlesdin et al., 1986; Young-Hoo et al., 2009).

3. Classification of high hip dislocation in adults

In the literature there are several classifications that determine high hip dislocation in adults. **Crowe** classification of hip dislocation describes four stages, depending on the position of the femoral head within the joint. The first three stages define the progressive migration of the head to the level of subluxation, while the fourth stage is luxation (Crowe et al., 1979).

According to the classification by **Eftekhar** the problem of the developmental disorders of the hip is viewed through acetabular changes. Four stages are also described; A/ slightly widened and dysplastic acetabulum with milder deformation of the head, B/ intermediately positioned false acetabulum, C/ high position of the false acetabulum, and D/ high non-weight bearing dislocation with the femoral head that has never been in contact with the iliac bone (Eftekhar 1978).

The most modern and up-to-now the best classification recommending total arthroplasty in relation to joint deficiency was given by **Hartofilakidis** et al. in 1996, according to which the condition was viewed as acetabular dysplasia, low dislocation and high dislocation (Hartofilakidis et al., 1996).

4. Treatment of high hip dislocation in adults

Treatment of the developmental disorder of the hip should be initiated at the moment of the disease detection, and the best results are achieved in the earliest childhood. At that period various forms of non-operative and operative treatments by biological surgeries are possible to be applied. (Vukasinovic & Djoric, 1994; Vukasinovic & Bascarevic, 2004). However, if the treatment is initiated only after the onset of arthrosis or under the conditions of high non-weight bearing hip luxation, operative treatment modalities are only reduced to total hip arthroplasty.

The operative procedure is most challenging because of changed anatomical correlations. The topographic correlation of muscles initiators of the hip, joint capsule and neurovascular elements are changed and unstable thus making the operative approach very difficult. The identification of bone structures, primarily of the true acetabulum, is also not at all easy (Lai et al., 1996, 2005; Charnley & Feagin 1973; Crowe et al., 1979; Dunn & Hess, 1976; Eskelinen et al., 2006; Hartofilakidis et al., 1998, 2004, 2008; Holinka et al., 2010; Paavilainen et al., 1990).

The ligamentum transversum is the only reliable parameter determining, not only the height and center of the artificial hip, but also the anteversion (flexion) position of the acetabular ring.

The proximal part of the femoral bone canal is very narrow, with markedly increased anteversion. The acetabular bone mass is underdeveloped, while the bone is insufficiently firm. The joint capsule is elongated, inelastic and thickened, while the surrounding muscles are without any strength, shortened and grown to the capsule. The neurovascular structures are shortened and dislocated from their anatomic positions (Carrlson et al., 2003; Holinka et al., 2010; Paavilainen et al., 1990).

In the past there were numerous unsuccessful attempts to perform total hip arthroplasty in adults at the location of high luxation caused by developmental disorder. Exactly due to excessively changed anatomic characteristics of the acetabulum and proximal femur, the operative procedure and the entire surgical concept are most complicated. Therefore, some authors consider high hip luxation as a contraindication for total arthroplasty (Figs. 1, 2, 3).

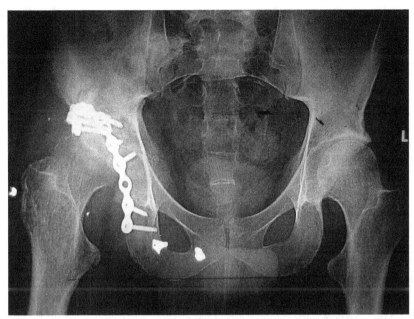

Fig. 1a. A 35-year old male after acetabular osteosynthesis performed due to traumatic dislocation of the right hip with superior and posterior acetabular wall fracture.

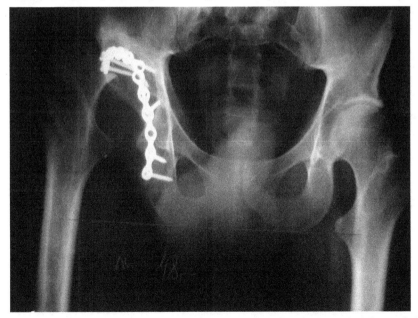

Fig. 1b. The same patient, six month later high dislocation of the hip occured due to failed osteosynthesis. Full absence of superior and posterior acetabular walls. Leg length discrepancy was 48 mm.

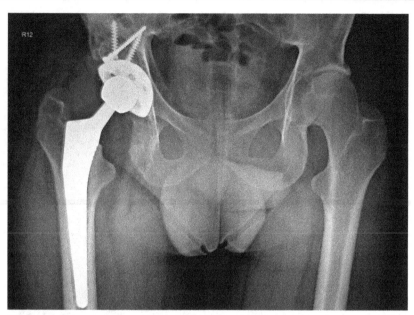

Fig. 1c. The same patient, three months after total arthroplasty of the hip, with the osteoplasty of the superior and posterior acetabular walls by solitary bone grafts from the bone bank. Restitution of leg length by positioning the acetabular component into the physiological hip rotation center.

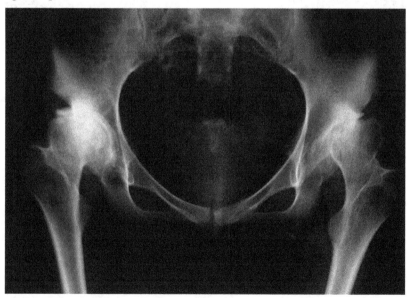

Fig. 2a. A 20-year old female with bilateral secondary arthrosis of the hips due to juvenile rheumatoid arthritis. Bilateral hip subluxation with various disorders of collo-diaphyseal femoral angle.

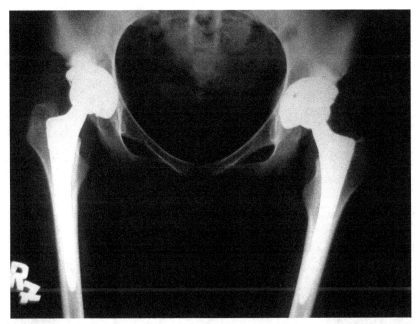

Fig. 2b. The same patient, one year after bilateral total arthroplasty of the hip with restitution of rotation centers.

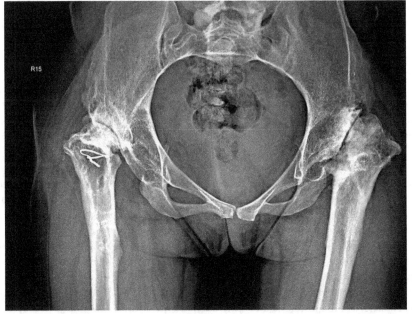

Fig. 3a. A 30-year old female with bilateral high dislocation of the hips after multiple surgeries due to neonatal sepsis.

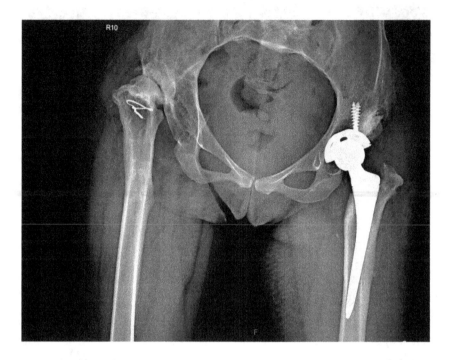

Fig. 3b. The same patient, one month after total arthroplasty of the left hip with restitution of rotation centers. The leg length equality is expected after the operation of the opposite hip.

4.1 Surgical procedures

The literature reports many operative techniques for total arthroplasty of the hip in patients with high dislocation. All agree on one point; the center of joint rotation should be restored, meaning that the acetabular component of the implant must be positioned in the primary paleo-acetabulum. This is the only way to expect good joint function, being the only mode to establish the physiological distance between the ends of the muscular initiators of hip motion, thus enabling their full strength. However, there is no full agreement as to the preparation and positioning of the proximal femur at the required level of the primary acetabulum (Carrlson et al., 2003; Crowe et al., 1979; Dunn & Hess, 1976; Eskelinen et al., 2006; Hartofilakidis et al., 1996, 1998, 2004; Holinka et al., 2010; Lai et al., 1996, 2005; Paavilainen et al., 1990).

Many surgical techniques have been described by authors discussing the type and modes of femoral abbreviation osteotomies. Some of them are performed through the very trochanteric mass (midtrochanteric), while others are done below it (subtrochanteric), with various forms of resection osteotomies with or without fixation of the proximal fragment or great trochanter. Some authors achieve the adequate position of the femur in correlation to paleo-acetabulum by extrafocal distraction after the resection of the joint. Arthroplasty is to follow as a new operative technique, where the entire operative procedure is performed in two acts. (Carrlson et al., 2003; Eskelinen et al., 2006; Hartofilakidis et al., 1996; Holinka et al., 2010; Lai et al., 1996, 2005; Paavilainen et al., 1990).

4.1.1 Total hip arthoplasty with iliofemoral distraction in high hip dislocation

As a part of total arthroplasty, the surgical technique applied to achieve the reduction of a high luxation of the hip without using femoral osteotomy is a relatively rare operative procedure. In the literature it was described by Lai et al. in 1996 and 2005, and then by Holinka et al. in 2010 (Carrlson et al., 2003; Eskelinen et al., 2006; Holinka et al., 2010; Lai et al., 1996, 2005).

The leading idea of this surgical procedure is based on the hypothesis that operative procedures with femoral abbreviation osteotomies, regardless of the type, could generally leave a considerable leg-length discrepancy, as well as muscular weakness of hip motion starters. The authors found a back-up for this notion in the articles by Crowe et al., Charnley et al., Dunn et al., Hartofilakidis et al., Paavilainen et al.Eskelinen et al., and others (Charnley & Feagin 1973; Crowe et al., 1979; Dunn & Hess, 1976; Eskelinen et al., 2006; Hartofilakidis et al., 1998; Paavilainen et al., 1990).

The operative procedure is performed in two acts. Namely, total arthroplasty is preceded by iliofemoral distraction with the Wagner's apparatus positioned in the ilium and distal femur. Before the distraction, it is necessary to perform subcutaneous adductor tenotomy of the hip, while femoral head resection with a total soft tissue release can be done before the distraction (Holinka et al.) or in the second act, as a part of total arthroplasty (Lai et al.). The distraction is performed gradually, 2-5 mm daily with regular X-ray check-ups and follow-up of neurocircular status of extremities, until the required joint reduction is achieved, bringing the femoral small trochanter into the acetabular teardrop level. During this period the patient is kept in bed. The second surgical act is performed after a few weeks involving removal of the Wagner's distraction apparatus and total arthroplasty of the hip.

The principles of total arthroplasty with positioning of the acetabular ring into the paleo-acetabulum and the stem in the femoral channel are standard. (Carrlson et al., 2003; Holinka et al., 2010; Lai et al., 1996, 2005; Paavilainen et al., 1990).

Such a surgical procedure is very complicated and requires long-term hospitalization and inactivity of the patient. The fact itself that in achieving the goal, total arthroplasty of the hip, requires two operative acts makes it twice riskier for the patient. In addition, the positioning of an extrafocal external apparatus in the area of the hip before arthroplasty might be as such problematic, because of exposing bone tissue to external environment over a long period of time. Strong Schantz screws in the femoral diaphysis can also present areas of decreased biomechanical resistance, particularly as known that the femur is anyway dysplastic in high luxations. Problems can also arise intraoperatively if there is extensive femoral anteversion. Namely, the positioning of a stem of standard geometry under such conditions could prove impossible to perform in the correction of overextensive anteversion. A solution could found in using special stems of small dimensions and/or modular geometry; however, this does not solve the problem of the residual anterior torsion of the femoral neck.

All this is probably the reason why such operative procedure is rarely described in the literature.

4.1.2 Total hip arthoplasty with femoral abbreviation osteotomies

Today there are basically two operative techniques for total arthroplasty of the hip in high luxations with femoral abbreviation osteotomies, and both are based on osteotomies in the subtrochanteric region.

One technique involves resection of a larger part of the trochanter mass, hence the entire metaphysis and a portion of diaphysis, with preservation of the great trochanter with abductor attachments, while by other operative procedures resection osteotomy is performed only on the diaphysis below the small trochanter, with the metaphysis remaining preserved.

Femoral abbreviation osteotomies in total arthroplasty of the hip, particularly when treating high luxations due to DDH, have been described by numerous authors (Dunn et al., 1976; Crowe et al., 1979 ; Paavilainen at al., 1990, 1993; Hartofilakidis et al., 1996, 1998, 2004, 2008 ; Papagelopoulos et al., 1996; Numair et al., 1997; Carrlson et al., 2003).

The original operative technique by Paavilainen et al. has been slightly modified by Carlsson et al., but basic postulates have remained the same. After exposing the hip through the posterolateral approach, abbreviation osteotomy of the proximal femur is performed at two levels, horizontal and sagittal. The diaphysis is osteotomized transversally 7-9 cm below the top of the great trochanter, and then osteotomy of the proximal fragment at the sagittal level is performed, thus leavening abductor attachments of the hip, primarily of the gluteus medius in the lateral part, which basically represents the great trochanter. The remaining portion of the proximal fragment is removed, i.e. if necessary it can be used as a graft. The conical stem of small dimensions is implanted into the distal fragment, namely directly into the femoral diaphysis. After having positioned the acetabular component of the endoprosthesis, the remaining proximal fragment is lowered onto the proximal portion of the diaphysis and fixed with screws and/or wire serclages. Walking with partial weight-bearing is immediately allowed, while full weight-bearing can be allowed after two months (Paavilainen at al., 1990, 1993; Carrlson et al., 2003).

This operative procedure has the advantage over those described above primarily because arthroplasty of the hip is performed in one act. Hospital stay is much shorter, with more rapid rehabilitation and without any significant limitation as to weight-bearing. Although osteotomy of the proximal femur is done, the function of the gluteus medius remains preserved. Rather, its strength is reinstituted with the distalization of the trochanter attachments.

Theoretically, the problem of this operative procedure might be non-healing of the great trochanter dislocated onto the diaphysis, however, authors have reported no such incidence in any of the cases. Also, theoretically, a delayed problem of potential revisional surgery might present a full loss of the metaphyseal bone of the proximal femur. The necessity to use a slightly more specific dysplastic stems, i.e. the impossibility of standard femoral implants (due to absent metaphyseal) does not present a true problem if taken into consideration a relatively small number of patients with such a condition.

At the Institute of Orthopaedic Surgery "Banjica" in Belgrade, high dislocation of the hip in adults is treated by transverse subtrochanteric abbreviational femoral osteotomy and, of course, a mandatory implantation of the acetabular component into the primary acetabulum. The operative technique was developed in 1984, however, over the time it has undergone minor modifications. The essence has remained identical, only some details were changed regarding the extent of capsular excision and the mode of femoral osteotomy. Namely, today we do not excise the entire joint capsule, although it is cautiously prepared and freed from attached muscles, while the stability of the femoral segments is achieved by the adapted transverse osteotomy and implantation of the standard stem with distal rotational stability. Also, over the last 11 years, with the emergence of new implants, above all hemispheric press-fit acetabular rings, the need for acetabuloplasty, which was almost regularly applied at the time of screw ring usage, nowadays is almost nonexistent (Radojevic & Zlatic, 1990; Tabak et al., 2003; Zlatic et al., 1990).

The relaxation of the neuromuscular elements is achieved by the postoperative positioning of the leg with the hip and the knee in flexion which is individually adapted to each patient. Gradual stretching is done during the next days and last on average for 2-3 days. Only then the patient is allowed to stand up and to begin walking. Individually tolerant weight bearing on the operated leg is immediately allowed. Discarding the crutches is also done on individual basis, above all depending on the patient's capability to achieve a stabile weight bearing within a given time. Certainly, osteotomy bone consolidation and the incorporation of endoprosthetic components also contribute to the decision on when walking supports could be discarded. Thromboembolic profilactic therapy is applied with low molecular weight heparine from the day of surgery until elapsed 35 postsurgical days (Fig. 4).

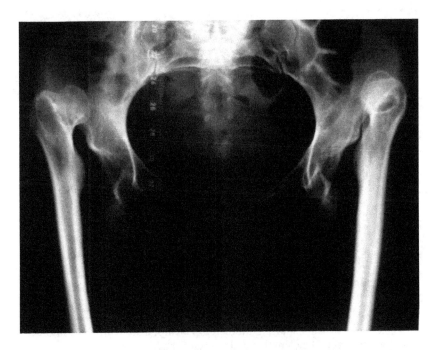

Fig. 4a. A 35-year old female with bilateral high dislocation of the hips due to DDH.

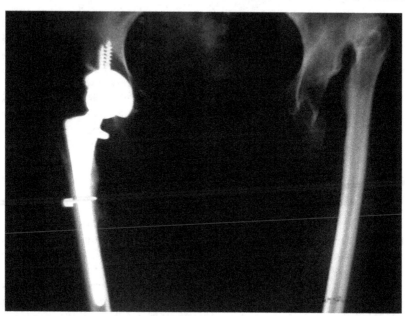

Fig. 4b. The same patient, nine months after total arthroplasty of the right hip. Good bone consolidation after four centimetres shortening subtrochanteric osteotomy.

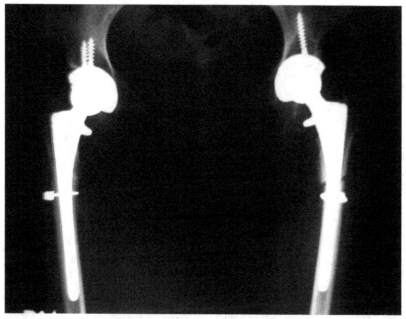

Fig. 4c. The same patient, three months after left hip arthroplasty with abreviation subtrochanteric osteotomy. Leg length equality established. Bone consolidation in progress, femoral stem stable.

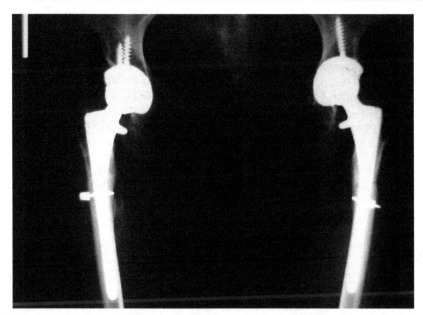

Fig. 4d. The same patient, 18 months after right total hip arthroplasty and nine month after left total hip artroplasty. Both osteotomies were fully consolidated.

5. Conclusion

As can be seen, all previously described operative techniques for high hip luxation treatment with total hip arthroplasty are reliable in hands of experienced surgeons.

According to our opinion both operative techniques with femoral abbreviation osteotomies have significant advantages over two-act operative procedures. The theoretical advantage of the latter described operative technique, with diaphyseal subtrochateric resection, over the former ones, with diaphyseal and metaphyseal resection, could be in the preservation of the bone metaphysis of the proximal femur with the possibility to use the standard midcoated implants without distal ingrowing and without additional fixation. On the other hand, the advantage of the former technique could refer to the healing of osteotomized fragments. Namely, a potentially delayed healing, and even non-healing of diaphyseal and metaphyseal bones in the subtrochanteric region is more probable than the fusion of firmly fixed great trochanter to the diaphysis.

6. Acknowledgment

This work was supported by Ministry of Education and Science, Republic of Serbia (Grant No. 41004).

7. References

Ando, M, Gotoh, E. (1990). Significance of inguinal folds for diagnosis of congenital dislocation of the hip in infants aged three to four mounts. *J Pediatr Orthop*, Vol. 10, No. 3, (May-Jun 1990) pp. (331-334), ISSN 0271-6798

Bascarevic Z, Vukasinovic Z, Slavkovic N, Dulic B, Trajkovic G, Bascarevic V, Timotijevic S. (2010). Alumina on alumina ceramic versus metal-on-highly cross-linked polyethylene bearings in total hip arthoplasty: a comparative study. *Int Orthop*, Vol. 34, No. 8, (November 2009) pp. (1129-1135), ISSN 0341-2695

Bascarevic, Z, Vukasinovic, Z. (2004). Diseases of the adult hip, In: *Special orthopaedics*, Vukasinovic, Z, pp. (275-303), Institute for orthopaedic diseases "Banjica" Belgrade, ISBN 86-82411-04-0, Belgrade

Besset, B, Fassier, F, Tanzer, M, Brooks, C. (2003). Total hip arthroplasty in patients younger than 21 years: a minimum 10 year follow up. *Can J Surg*, Vol. 46, No. 4, (August 2003), pp. (257-262), ISSN 1488-2310

Betz, R, Cooperman, D, Wopperer, J. (1990). Late sequelae of septic arthritis of the hip in infancy and childhood. *Je Pediatr Orthop*, Vol.10, No. 3, (May-Jun 1990), pp. (365-372), ISSN 0271-6798

Carrlson, A, Bjorkman, A, Ringsberg, K, Schewelov, T. (August 2003). Untreated congenital and posttraumatic high dislocation of the hip treated by replacement in adult age. *Acta Orthop Scand*, Vol. 74, No. 4, (August 2003), pp. (389-396), ISSN 0001-6470

Charnley, J, Feagin, JA. (1973). Low-friction arthroplasty in congenital subluxation of the hip. *Clin Orthop Relat Res*, Vol. 91, No. 3-4, (March-April 1973), pp. (98-113), ISSN 0009-921X

Cherney, D, Westin, G. (1989). Acetabular development in the infants dislocated hips. *Clin Orthop Relat Res*, Vol. 242, No. 5, (May 1989), pp. (98-103), ISSN 0009-921X

Choi IH, Pizzutillo PD, Bowen JR, Dragann R, Malhis T. (1990). Sequelae and reconstruction after septic arthritis of the hip in infants. *J Bone Joint Surg Am*, Vol. 72, No. 8, (September 1990), pp. (1150-1165), ISSN 0021-9355

Crowe, JF, Mani, VJ, Ranawat, CS. (1979). Total hip replacement in congenital dislocation and dysplasia of the hip. *J Bone Joint Surg Am*, Vol. 61, No. 1, (January 1979), pp. (15-23), ISSN 0021-9355

Delimar, D, Cicak, N, Klobucar, H, Pecina, M, Korzinek, K. (2002). Acetabular roof reconstruction with pedicled iliac graft. *Int Orthop*, Vol. 26, No. 6, (July 2002), pp. (344-348), ISSN 0341-2695

Dunn, HK, Hess, WE. (1976). Total hip reconstruction in chronically dislocated hips. *J Bone Joint Surg Am*, Vol. 58, No. 6, (September 1976), pp. (838-845), ISSN 0021-9355

Eftekhar, NS. (1978). *Principles of total hip arthroplasty*, CV Mosby, ISBN 0306439921, St. Louis

Eskelinen, A, Helenius, I, Remes, V, Ylinen, P, Talloroth, K, Paavilainen, T. (2006). Cementless total hip arthroplasty in patients with high congenital hip dislocation. *J Bone Joint Surg Am*, Vol. 88, No. 1, (January 2006), pp. (80-91), ISSN 0021-9355

Hartofilakidis, G, Georgiades, G, Babis, GC, Yiannakopoulos, CK. (2008). Evaluation of two surgical techniques for acetabular reconstruction in total hip replacement for congenital hip disease: results after a minimum ten-year follow-up. *J Bone Joint Surg Br*, Vol. 90, No. 6, (June 2008), pp. (724-730), ISSN 0301-620X

Hartofilakidis, G, Karachalios, T. (2004). Total hip arthroplasty for congenital hip disease. *J Bone Joint Surg Am*, Vol. 86-A, No. 2, (February 2004), pp. (242-250), ISSN 0021-9355

Hartofilakidis, G, Stamos, K, Karachalios, T. (1998). Treatment of high dislocation of the hip in adults with total hip arthroplasty. Operative technique and long-term clinical results. *J Bone Joint Surg Am*, Vol. 80, No. 4, (April 1998), pp. (510-517), ISSN 0021-9355

Hartofilakidis, G, Stamos, K, Karachalios, T, Ioannidis, TT, Zacharakis, N. (1996). Congenital hip disease in adults. Classification of acetabular deficiencies and operative treatment with acetabuloplasty combined with total hip arthroplasty. *J Bone Joint Surg Am*, Vol. 78, No. 5, (May 1996), pp. (683-92), ISSN 0021-9355

Holinka, J, Pfeiffer, M,Hofstaetter, JG, Lass, R, Kotz, RI, Giurea, A. (2010). Total hip replacement in congenital high hip dislocation following iliofemoralmonotube distraction. *Int Orthop*, Vol. 35, No. 5, (March 2010), pp. (639-645), ISSN 0341-2695

Klisic, P. (1989). Congenital dislocation of the hip: a misleading term. *J Bone Joint Surg*, Vol. 71, No. 1, (January 1989), pp. (136-139), ISSN 0301-620X

Klisic, P, Rakic, D, Pajic, D. (1984). Triple prevention of congenital dislocation of the hip. *J Pediatr Orthop*, Vol. 4, No. 6, (November 1984), pp. (759-761), ISSN 0271-6798

Lai, KA, Liu, J, Liu, TK. (1996). Use of iliofemoral distraction in reducing high congenital dislocation of the hip before total hip arthroplasty. *J Arthoplasty*, Vol.11, No. 5, (August 1996), pp. (588-593), ISSN 0883-5403

Lai, KA, Shen, WJ, Huang, LW, Chen, MY. (2005). Cementless total hip arthroplasty and limb-length equalization in patients with unilateral Crowe type-IV hip dislocation. *J Bone Joint Surg Am*, Vol. 87, No. 2, (February 2005), pp. (339-345), ISSN 0021-9355

Learmonth, ID, Heywood, AW, Kaye, J, Dall, D. (1989). Radiological loosening after cemented hip replacement for juvenile chronic arthritis. *J Bone Joint Surg Br*, Vol. 71, No. 2, (March 1989), pp. (45-55), ISSN 0301-620X

Maric, Z, Haynes, RJ. (1993). Total hip arthroplasty in juvenile rheumatoid arthritis. *Clin Orthop*, Vol. 290, No. 5, (May 1993), pp. (197-199), ISSN 0009-921X

Numair, J, Joshi, AB, Murphy, JC, Porter, ML, Hardinge, K. (1997). Total hip arthroplasty for congenital dysplasia or dislocation of the hip. Survivorship analysis and long-term results. *J Bone Joint Surg Am*, Vol. 79, No. 9, (September 1997), pp. (1352–1360), ISSN 0021-9355

Paavilainen, T, Hoikka, V, Solonen, KA. (1990). Cementless total replacement for severely dysplastic or dislocated hips. *J Bone Joint Surg Br*, Vol. 72, No. 2, (March 1990), pp. (205–211), ISSN 0301-620X

Papachristou, G, Hatzigrigoris, P, Panousis, K, Plessas, S, Sourlas, J, Levidiotis, C, Chronopoulos, E. (2006). Total hip arthroplasty for developmental hip dysplasia. *Int Orthop*, Vol. 30, No. 1, (February 2006), pp. (21–25), ISSN 0341-2695

Papagelopoulos, P, Trousdale, RT, Lewallen, DG. (1996). Cementless total hip arthroplasty with femoral osteotomy for proximal femoral deformity. *Clin Orthop*, Vol. 332, No. 11, (November 1996), pp. (151-162), ISSN 0009-921X

Pitto, RP, Schikora, N. (2004). Acetabular reconstruction in developmental hip dysplasia using reinforcement ring with a hook. *Int Orthop*, Vol. 28, No. 4, (August 2004), pp. (202–205), ISSN 0341-2695

Radojevic, B, Zlatic, M. (1990). An L-shaped bone graft for acetabular deficiency. *J Bone Joint Surg Br*, Vol. 72, No. 1, (January 1990), pp. (152-153), ISSN 0301-620X

Ruddlesdin, C, Ansell, BM, Arden, GP, Swann, M. (1986). Total hip replacement in children with juvenile chronic arthritis. *J Bone Joint Surg Br*, Vol. 68, No. 2, (March 1986), pp. (218-222), ISSN 0301-620X

Tabak, AY, Celebi, L, Muratli, H, Yagmurlu, F, Aktekin, C, Bicimoglu, A. (2003). Cementless total hip replacement in patients with high total dislocation: the results of femoral shortening by subtrochanteric segmental resection. *Acta Orthop Traumatol Turc*, Vol. 37, No.4, (April 2003), pp. (277-283), ISSN 1017-995x

Vukasinovic, Z, Bascarevic, Z. (2004). Diseases of the infant hip, In: *Special orthopaedics*, Vukasinovic Z, pp (237-273), Institute for orthopaedic diseases "Banjica" Belgrade, ISBN 86-82411-04-0, Belgrade

Vukasinovic, Z, Djoric, I. (1994). Developmental disorder of the hip, In: *Hip diseases in childhood*, Vukasinovic Z, pp. (37-78), Special orthopeadic hospital „Banjica" Belgrade, ISBN 86-82411-01-6, Belgrade

Kim YH, Seo HS, Kim JS. (2009). Outcomes after THA in patients with high hip after childhood sepsis. *Clin Orthop Relat Res*, Vol. 467, No. 9, (September 2009), pp. (2371-2378), ISSN 0009-921X

Zlatic, M, Radojevic, B, Lazovic, C. (1990). Reconstruction of the hipoplastyc acetabulum in cementless arthroplasty of the hip. *Int Orthop*,Vol. 14, No.4, (April 1990), pp. (371-375), ISSN 0341-2695

12

Modular Femoral Neck Fracture After Total Hip Arthroplasty

Igor Vučajnk and Samo K. Fokter
Celje General and Teaching Hospital
Slovenia

1. Introduction

In the middle of the 20th century total hip arthroplasty (THA) became the most popular and the most common reconstructive procedure of the hip. It is important as a last resort in treatment of terrible pain due to progressive hip arthritis of different etiologies. Implanting an artificial hip prosthesis, the surgeon helps the patient by releasing the pain and restoring the range of movement so that the patient can resume his normal activities.

Historically, treatment of progressive osteoarthritis evolved from arthrodesis through different osteotomies, nerve divisions, joint debridements, and interpositions of different organic or inorganic materials between the articular surfaces, towards the final introduction of total hip endoprosthesis. The first endoprostheses were made of glass. Afterwards the quality of the materials progressed from plastic, steel, to cobalt-chromium alloys and finally titanium alloys. Additionally, considerable effort was made to improve the manufacturing techniques, hip biomechanics and the usage of appropriate materials (Harkess & Crockarell, 2007). The studies of materials revealed that orthopaedic implants must be biocompatible; they have to resist all forms of corrosion (Sharan, 1999), resist degradation and withstand all forces that potentially apply. Different designs of total hip endoprostheses follow different philosophies. Two kinds of prosthesis designs are currently used in primary hip arthroplasty. Monoblock is a femoral stem prosthesis made of a single piece, while modular prostheses are made of two modules: the femoral stem and the femoral neck. The stem can be of different sizes, and the neck is of different sizes and different neck angle versions.

According to the American Academy of Orthopaedic Surgeons (AAOS), more than 193,000 total hip replacements are performed yearly in the United States alone. The prediction for the US is that the number of total hip replacements will at least double by the year 2030 (Wilson N., 2008).

2. Modular neck hip prosthesis

Modular neck hip prosthesis has been gaining popularity worldwide for the last thirty years. Modular stems are commonly used in revision hip surgery. The use of this kind of endoprosthesis was first published in 1948 by McBride, then later by Bousquet and Bornard in 1978. Several companies presently offer different versions of modular neck hip endoprostheses for primary total hip arthroplasty (Keppler, 2006). The advantage of this type of endoprosthesis is that the surgeon has an intraoperative choice of neck version and neck length independently of the stem size. The surgeon can then adjust the femoral offset, correct leg length and achieve hip stability.

Modular hip endoprostheses can be classified as proximal, mid-stem, distal and multi-modular. The proximal ones have modules for sleeve, shoulder and neck, neck, collars and proximal pads (Froehlich, 2006). In this chapter we focus on proximal modular neck endoprostheses.

Important differences exist between the two sexes in femoral neck length, femoral shaft diameter, collum-caput-diaphysis angle (CCD), neck version and offset (Traina, 2009). In order to properly restore the hip biomechanics these parameters must be kept in mind. Appropriate restoration of femoral offset and appropriate soft tissue balancing is necessary. Unsatisfactory restoration of hip biomechanics can and will lead to limping, abductor muscle imbalances, and higher rates of wearing. In order to achieve the best biomechanics of the reconstructed hip, preoperative planning is essential. However, as the femoral version cannot be appropriately and adequately assessed with standard radiographs, modular hip prosthesis offers some advantage during the operation. In addition, some benefits of modular neck hip prosthesis in developmental dysplasia of the hip (DDH) have been reported. One study showed that monoblock stems restore offset in only one out of three patients. Eight different neck shaft angle solutions are necessary to restore the anatomy in 50% of the patients (Massin, 2000).

3. Complications associated with modular neck hip prosthesis

The complications associated with modular neck hip arthroplasty are divided in medical complications and complications associated with surgery and materials. Medical complications, such as cardiovascular, thromboembolic, pulmonary, anaemic and renal complications as well as delirium can be prevented or at least minimized with careful preoperative risk assessment and proper perioperative care (Foerg, 2005). Other complications including joint infection, nerve and blood vessel injury, and bleeding during or after the surgery can be reduced by proper operative techniques. Leg length inequality, prosthesis dislocation, and prosthesis impingement can be prevented with a proper choice of offset and neck version. The highly corrosive environment of the human body demands the use of such biomaterials which will withstand degradation that could lead to another serious complication – failure of the prosthetic material.

Instability is the second most common complication after aseptic loosening (Abraham, 2005). Dislocation rates vary among reports from 0.5% to 11%. The risk of dislocation is associated with time from the operation and with traumatic events, polyethylene wear and pseudocapsule laxity.

4. Prosthesis size and materials

Modular neck hip endoprostheses are made of different numbers of modules. The prosthesis used for primary THA is made of two modules, the femoral stem and the femoral modular neck. The femoral stem comes in different sizes in order to fit different femoral dimensions. The numbers of stem sizes differ from one manufacturer to the other. The femoral neck comes in different sizes and versions as well, and the number again depends on the manufacturer. The two modules connect at the stem neck junction called the taper. The modularity gives important advantage for fine adjustments of leg length and femoral anteversion.

The materials used for modular femoral stem and modular neck are made of cobalt alloys (Co-Cr-Mo; cobalt-chromium-molybdenum) and of titanium alloys (Ti-6Al-4V; titanium-aluminium-vanadium). Cobalt alloys are among the strongest materials used for implants and can resist high-loading. The added molybdenum increases the strength even more. Chromium is added for hardness and makes the alloy more resistant to corrosion. The unique property of titanium alloys is their tissue biocompatibility. Corrosion is very limited in titanium alloys and they resist to crevice corrosion because they form a passive layer of oxide films (titanium oxide) on their surface. The biomaterials used have to resist crevice corrosion, fretting corrosion, galvanic corrosion, and pitting corrosion in order to withstand the degradation process. Also, the materials must have proper mechanical and wear properties.

5. Modular neck fracture

An increasing number of recently published case reports and studies describe catastrophic failures of modular femoral neck prostheses resulting from material fracture. The Swedish Hip Arthroplasty Register Annual Report of femoral hip stems noted overall femoral stem implant failure in 493 prostheses out of the 299,368 primary hip arthroplasties performed from 1979 to 2008 (1.4%) (Garellick et al., 2009). A report on the Metha Short Hip Stem Prosthesis (Aesculap AG, Tuttlingen, Germany) also showed a 1.4% failure rate of modular necks (68 neck failures out of 5000 THA) (Grupp, 2010). According to the Wright Company, the Profemur (Profemur Z, Wright Medical Technology, Inc., Arlington, TN, USA) modular neck fracture rate in 198,331 implanted endoprostheses has been calculated to 0.028% (Wright Medical Technology Inc., 2010). The Profemur world wide fracture rate in all necks, including long and short necks is reported to be 0.058% (6 fractures out of every 10,000 THA) (Wright Medical Technology Inc., 2010). Both in Wright and in Aesculap, the necks were made of titanium alloys. This complication is supposed to occur in almost all cases with long necks, heavier patients and male patients. Both studies concluded that titanium long necks should be replaced with cobalt chrome alloy necks because they are safer (Wright Medical Technologies Inc., 2010; Grupp, 2010). The Zimmer Company reviewed over 300,000 primary VerSys prostheses (VerSys Hip System, Zimmer Inc., Warsaw, IN, USA) implanted since the year 2000 and their fracture rate was less than 0.0018% (Hertzler et al., 2009). A center implanting Acumatch M-series cementless hip endoprostheses (Acumatch M-series, Exactech Inc., Gainesville, Florida, USA) reported on fracture rates of 1.6% (8 fractures out of 500 implanted prostheses) (Paliwal, 2010).

There are many reasons for prosthesis fracture. As mentioned in the previous section, orthopaedic implants are subject to crevice corrosion, fretting corrosion, galvanic corrosion and pitting corrosion (Sharan, 1999). The changing demographics of the patients undergoing total hip replacement surgeries could also contribute to the fracture rates. These include increased patient weight, increased physical activities, increased life expectancy, and the timing of the operation (Chrowninshield, 2006).

Fretting is a phenomenon which occurs between two contacting bodies experiencing reciprocating motion. In our case small scale reciprocating movements occur between the femoral stem and the femoral neck at the taper junction. When the main factor causing fretting is oxidation the process is called fretting corrosion. The more the neck is in varus position and the longer the neck is, the greater is the tendency for fretting because of the increased lever arm. Microscopic cracks develop in the fretting zone that can lead to femoral neck fracture. Studies in vitro show that mechanical loading accelerates the corrosion process (Goldberg and Gilbert, 2002).

Another type of process occurring at the taper connection is crevice corrosion. The crevice between two modules will be a corrosion site if there is enough space to allow the income of an aqueous solution (Colliere et al., 1992). The crevice should be sufficiently narrow to maintain a stagnant zone. As corrosion in this zone progresses, oxygen depletion will lead to an excess of positively charged ions in the surrounding aqueous environment of the crevice. The negatively charged chloride ions will migrate to balance them. As a result, hydrochloric acid will form. Hydrochloric acid can dissolve titanium or cobalt alloys which are otherwise stable. Once the crevice corrosion has begun it continues even in the absence of loading.

Concern was raised in the past that galvanic corrosion can arise from inappropriate combinations of dissimilar metal components. Galvanic corrosion is an electrochemical process in which two physically connected dissimilar metals experience metallic deterioration while being exposed to electrically conductive fluids. Different metals have different electrochemical characteristics. When two dissimilar metals are placed together, electrons will start to flow spontaneously from one metal to the other. The loss of electrons from the active metal is called oxidation and oxidation will lead to the process of corrosion (Shetty, 1989). Corrosion will start the release of metal ions and will cause among other complications damage to the prosthesis surface. This can lead to the loss of material strength and eventually to failure.

There is also a form of extremely localized, symmetric corrosion called pitting corrosion. It leads to the creation of small holes in the metal. The mechanism of pitting corrosion is probably the same as crevice corrosion.

The studies of modular neck adapters and stems showed that fretting leads to microcracks on the surface (Grupp, 2010; Wright Medical Technologies Inc., 2010). Fretting is accompanied with crevice corrosion and pitting corrosion. As mentioned above, the passive oxide film formed in titanium alloys is permanently destroyed by fretting corrosion and crevice corrosion. Fretting reduces the fatigue strength of titanium alloys. Fretting at the connection can be increased by the intraoperative contamination of taper with small particles of bone or tissue. Contamination should always be prevented by assembling the device carefully and drying the components before the assembly (Grupp, 2010). Both studies concluded that the change of femoral neck material from titanium alloys to cobalt alloys increases the safety of the connection (Grupp, 2010; Wright Medical Technologies Inc., 2010). Cobalt alloys have the same fatigue strength, they form the passive oxide layer and have excellent fretting corrosion characteristics in comparison to titanium alloys. Cobalt alloys are superior in stiffness and modules of elasticity, notch sensitivity, crack propagation, and abrasion compared to titanium alloys. However, cobalt alloys are inferior to titanium alloys in characteristics of crevice corrosion and are more allergenic. The authors recommended that heavier patients, especially those weighing more than 100 kg, and more physically active male patients require long necks made of cobalt alloys.

Froehlich et al. did a follow up of their experience with seven different modular stems implanted since 1984 (Froehlich, 2006). They implanted 2,248 stems for primary THA in cemented and uncemented way. They used S-Rom (S-Rom Modular Hip System, JMPC/DePuy, Warsaw, IN, USA), Apex Modular (Apex Modular Hip System, Global Orthopaedic Technology, Unanderra, NSW, Australia), K2 Apex (Apex K2 Modular Hip System, Omni Life Science, Inc., East Taunton, MA, USA), OTI/Encore R-120 cemented stem, OTI/Encore R-120 porous c.c. cementless stem (R-120 Modular Stem, DJO Surgical, Austin, TX, USA), UniSyn (UniSyn Total Hip System, Hayes Medical, Inc., El Dorado Hills, CA, USA) and Cremascoli Modular Neck (Wright Medical Technologies, Inc., Arlington, TN, USA). They experienced 12 femoral component failures, 2 in a c.c. proximal modular neck and 10 in proximal modular titanium shoulder neck. The authors remain enthusiastic about modularity and continue to use modular stems in their practice. The reason for failure in their cases was a single high load event and suggested quasi-static shear failure of the pin alignment. The OTI/Encore modular neck failure occurred in the distal neck engagement taper (Froehlich, 2006). The company increased the upper taper diameter, the lower taper diameter, the surface area, and the distal taper length so that the fatigue testing results improved.

Several recent case reports exist describing the failure of modular necks of the Profemur prostheses (Profemur Z, Wright Medical Technologies Inc., Arlington, TN, USA) (Atwood, 2010; Wright G., 2010; Wilson D. J., 2010). They describe a well integrated implant that could only be removed with trochanteric osteotomy. Usually the initiation site for failure was the anterior and superior part of the neck. Degradation of the polished surface was noted at the insertion point of the taper. Also, evidence of abrasion and corrosion was seen (Dangles, 2010). The Federal Drug Administration Manufacturer and User Facility Device Experience (FDA MAUDE) database describes 98 adverse effects for the Profemur modular neck prosthesis for the years 2000-2009. 37 of those include breakage of the femoral neck (FDA MAUDE, as cited in Skendzel et al., 2011). Skendzel et al. reported on two cases of fractured Profemur modular neck and concluded that the long varus necks used increased the bending moment by 32.7% when compared to short varus necks (Skendzel et al., 2011). The stress was concentrated at the modular junction. Removal of the complete femoral component was required during revision surgery because the Morse taper could not be removed. Both patients experienced a traumatic event before the failure. Atwood et al. described the fracture of a Profemur long straight neck in a man of 2 m height and 109.8 kg weight who fell on his hip (Atwood, 2010). The surgery revealed a crack of 2 mm below the stem edge. They found the initiation site near the lateral-anterior corner of the neck. They also found signs of crevice corrosion and fretting wear.

Grupp et al. studied the Metha Short Hip Stem Prosthesis (Metha Short Hip Stem Prosthesis, Aesculap AG, Tuttlingen, Germany) as a consequence of several reports of failed titanium alloy femoral necks (Grupp, 2010). Out of 5,000 THA they found 68 neck adapter failures. They found neither processing or material deviation nor incorrect dimensioning. The retrieved prostheses showed a similar fracture pattern with the fracture starting in the anterolateral area at the upper part of the cone where there is maximum biomechanical stress. The reason for failure was attributed to fretting, fretting corrosion, and crevice corrosion which lead to the loss of fatigue strength of titanium alloy. The combination of factors listed above, as well as contamination of the cone adapter with fluids or particles, increased patient weight, high activity level, male gender, and CCD angle of 135 and smaller increased the rate of failure. They concluded that the change to cobalt-based alloy modular necks increases the safety of cone connection.

However, some studies did not show any problems regarding modular femoral components. The study by Toni et al. showed no clinical complications related to modular necks (Toni et al., 2001). They studied 216 hip prostheses of AnCA Fit type (AnCA Fit, Cremascoli Ortho, Milan, Italy) which were implanted from June 1995 to December 1997. Another study by Duwelius et al. using the Zimmer M/L Taper Hip Prosthesis with Kinectiv Technology (Zimmer M/L Taper Hip Prosthesis with Kinectiv Technology, Zimmer, Warsaw, IN, USA) on 634 patients from April 2007 to November 2008 showed no complications related to modular neck failure (Duwelius et al., 2010). The stem and neck were manufactured from titanium alloy (Ti6Al4V).

6. Case report

At the Depatment of Orthopaedic Surgery and Sports Trauma, Celje General and Teaching Hospital, Celje, Slovenia, modular hip prostheses have been used since the year 1992 in selected patients. The first prosthesis used was GSP (Cremascoli Ortho, Sorem Ortho, Toulon, France) and at the time of writing the prosthesis in use is the Profemur Z (Wright Medical Technology, Inc., Arlington, TN, USA). From 1992 to 2008, 306 modular neck hip prostheses of three different types were implanted at our department. From 1992 to 2004, 88 GSP modular neck hip prostheses (Cremascoli Orthopaedics, Sorem Ortho, Toulon, France) were implanted. From 2002 to 2006 we implanted 58 Anca Dual Fit hip stems (Cremascoli Ortho, Milan, Italy). In 2006 we started implanting Profemur Z modular neck hip prostheses (Wright Medical Technology, Inc., Arlington, TN, USA) and 160 of these were implanted by the end of 2008.

In December 2010, a 69-year old male was admitted to our hospital's emergency department with acute pain in his right hip. The pain appeared after a fall on his right side from standing height. The examination revealed right inguinal tenderness and shortening of his right lower extremity with external rotation. The review of standard radiographic exams showed modular prosthesis neck fracture. This was the first such complication seen at our department (Fig. 1). The patient's height was 178 cm and he weighed 110 kg (BMI 34.7). He was treated at our institution in 1998 when he was 56 years old. At that time his BMI was 31.6 (weight 100 kg). The operation was performed because the patient suffered from rheumatoid arthritis with the involvement of his right hip. A fully modular cementless total hip endoprosthesis was implanted (fully hidroxy-apatite coated femoral stem (GSP) with modular cobalt-chromium long straight neck, 28 mm diameter ceramic head, and acetabulum of the press-fit type (ANCA-Fit) with ceramic acetabular insert, (Cremascoli Orthopaedics, Sorem Ortho, Toulon, France). None of the postoperative visits or radiographic exams showed any signs of wear or other complications. The patient was pain free before the event.

Revision surgery was scheduled as soon as we received the custom made acetabular cup inlay (ANCA-Fit, Wright Medical Technology Inc., Arlington, TN, USA). The operation was performed by the same surgeon and the previous lateral approach was used. Revision surgery confirmed the fracture of the modular prosthesis neck. It was impossible to remove only the remaining neck from the taper, so that the entire femoral stem had to be removed. The femoral stem was well integrated in the femur and femoral osteotomy was necessary in order to remove the implant. Macroscopically, the tissue showed no metal debris or granuloma. The remaining part of the fractured neck module was approximately 2 mm below the top of the taper (Fig. 2-4).

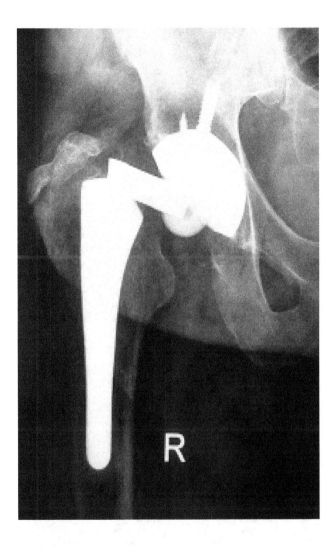

Fig. 1. Standard antero-posterior radiograph of the patient's right hip at admission.
(Courtesy M. Kotnik, M. D.)

In order to properly reconstruct the biomechanics of the hip, cementless revision modular stem with ceramic head (Waldemar Link GmbH & Co, Hamburg, Germany) was used. The acetabular lining was exchanged as well and a custom made ANCA-Fit (Wright Medical Technology, Inc., Arlington, TN, USA) component implanted (Fig. 5). Standard tissue specimens were collected during the revision procedure for microbiologic cultures which showed no bacterial growth.

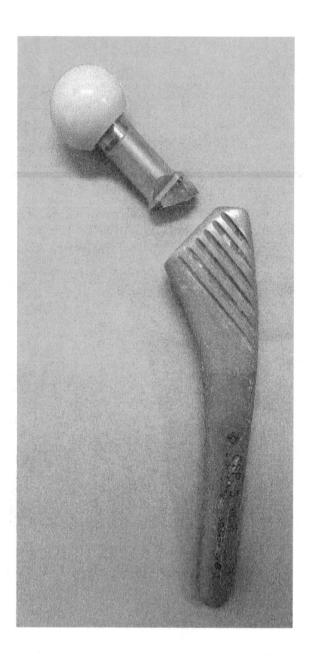

Fig. 2. Photograph of the retrieved fully-modular prosthesis showing the modular neck fracture.

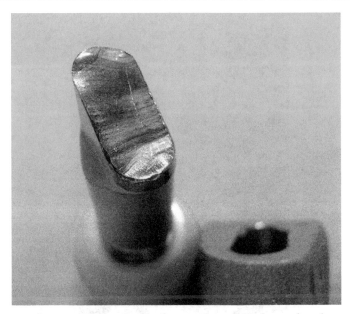

Fig. 3. A close-up photograph showing the fractured modular femoral neck.

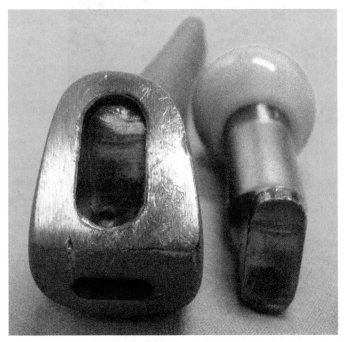

Fig. 4. Photograph showing the removed prosthesis with fractured neck and the remaining of the modular neck in the femoral stem taper.

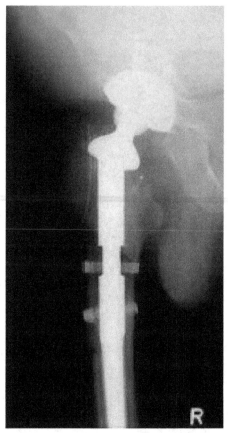

Fig. 5. Radiograph of the revised right hip with the cementless revision modular prosthesis in place. (Courtesy M. Kotnik, M. D.)

7. Conclusion

Modular neck hip prostheses are nowadays wildly used around the globe. The Profemur stem (Wright Medical Technology Inc., Arlington, TN, USA) only was sold in more than 200,000 units by the end of 2010 (Wright Medical Technologies Inc., 2010). There are many benefits in proximal modularity. The theoretical benefits of modular neck include bone and tissue conservation, restoration of joint biomechanics, reduced blood loss, easier rehabilitation, ease of revision, simple surgical technique, and different modular options (McTighe, 2008). In addition, the possibility of implanting a stem with a retroverted modular neck can prevent cup impingement and dislocation of the prosthesis. Moreover, if revision operation is necessary for the dislocated THA, only exchange of the modular neck might be required. The surgeon has an intraoperative option of choosing the appropriate neck length, neck version and CCD angle independently of the femoral stem size, taking into account the considerable differences in stem sizes between the two sexes (Traina, 2009). The proximal modular neck type of the prosthesis is useful in primary hip arthroplasty due to the significant differences among the individuals requiring hip reconstruction. Some types of modular neck prostheses offer as much as 60 different variations with modularity compared to only about 10 options offered by monoblock stems (Duwelius, 2010).

However, added modularity brings another possibility for complication. Recent reports emphasize the need for changing the neck material from titanium alloys to the safer cobalt-chromium alloys. Constant evaluation of laboratory material should be continued, even though it does not always guarantee proper information regarding in vivo parameters. Careful preoperative planning should be performed in spite of modular neck THA allowing anatomic reconstruction of the hip. The increased variety of intraoperative surgical options with the fully-modular stems should not be an excuse for bad surgical technique and improper cup position.

8. References

Abraham R. & Arthur L. M. (2005). Instability after Total Hip Replacement. *Seminars in Arthroplasty*, Vol.16, No.2, (June 2005), pp. 132-141, ISSN 1045-4527

American Academy of Orthopaedic Surgeons, AAOS. (April 2009). Total Hip Replacement, In: *Your orthopaedic connection*, Accessed June 23 2011, Available from: <http://orthoinfo.aaos.org/topic.cfm?topic=a00377>

Atwood, S.; Patten, E.; Bozic, K.; Pruitt, L. & Ries, M. (2010). Corrosion-induced fracture of a double-modular hip prosthesis: a case report. *The Journal of Bone and Joint Surgery*, Vol.92, No.6, (June 2010), pp. 1522-1525, ISSN 0021-9355

Collier, J.; Surprenant, V.; Jensen, R.; Mayor, M. & Surprenant, H. (1992). Corrosion between the components of modular femoral hip prostheses. *The Journal of Bone and Joint Surgery, British Volume*, Vol.74, No.4, (July 1992), pp. 511-517, ISSN 0301-620X

Crowninshield, R.; Rosenberg, A. & Sporer, S. (2006). Changing demographics of patients with total joint replacement. *Clinical Orthopaedics and Related Research*, Vol.443, No.2, (February 2006), pp. 266-272, ISSN 0009-921X

Dangles, C. J. & Altstetter, C. J. (2010). Failure of the modular neck in a total hip arthroplasty. *The Journal of Arthroplasty*, Vol.25, No.7, (October 2010), pp. 5-7, ISSN 0883-5403

Duwelius, P. J.; Hartzband, M. A.; Burkhart, R.; Carnahan, C.; Blair, S.; Wu, Y. & Grunkemeier, G. L. (2010). Clinical Results of a Modular Neck Hip System: Hitting the "Bull's-Eye" More Accurately. *American Journal of Orthopedics*, Vol.39, Suppl.10, (October 2010), pp. 2-6, ISSN 1078-4519

Foerg, F. (2005). Medical Complications Associated with Total Hip Arthroplasty. *Seminars in Arthroplasty*, Vol.16, No.2, (June 2005), pp. 88-99, ISSN 1045-4527

Froehlich, J. A.; McTighe, T.; Cameron, H. U.; Kegg, K.; Keggi, J.; Kennon, R. & Woodgate, I. (2006). Defining the Role of Modular Stem Designs in THA, *ITSA 19th Annual Symposium*, New York City, October 2006

Garellick, G.; Kärrholm, J.; Rogmark, C. & Herberts, P. (October 2009). Swedish Hip Arthroplasty Register Annual Report 2008, In: *Department of Ortopaedics, Faculty of Medicine, Göteborg University*, Accessed June 24 2011, Available from: <https://www.jru.orthop.gu.se/>

Goldberg, J. & Gilbert, J. (2002). In vitro corrosion testing of modular hip tapers. *Journal of Biomedical Materials Research, Part B, Applied Biomaterials*, Vol.64, No.2, (December 2002), pp. 78-93, ISSN 1552-4973

Grupp, T.; Weik, T.; Bloemer, W. & Knaebel, H. (2010). Modular titanium alloy neck adapter failures in hip replacement - failure mode analysis and influence of implant material. *BMC Musculoskeletal Disorders*, Vol.11, No.3, (January 2010), pp. 1-12

Harkess, J. W. & Crockarell, J. R. (2007). Arthroplasty of the hip, In: *Campbell's Operative Orthopaedics*, Canale, S. T. & Beaty, J. H., (Eds.), pp. 314-351, Mosby, An Imprint of Elsevier, Retrieved from <http://www.mdconsult.com/books/page.do?eid=4-u1.0-B978-0-323-03329-9..50010-6&isbn=978-0-323-03329-9&uniqId=263852506-2#4-u1.0-B978-0-323-03329-9..50010-6>

Hertzler, J. S.; Johnson, T. S. & Meulink, S. L. (2009). *Performance evaluation of Kinectiv™ Technology*, Zimmer, Inc, Retrieved from <http://www.zimmer.com/web/enUS/pdf/Performance_Evaluation_of_Kinectiv_Technology.pdf>

Keppler, L.; Cameron, H. U. & McTighe, T. (2006). The Role of Modularity in Primary THA - Is There One?, *AAOS Scientific Exhibit*, Chicago, 2006

Massin, P.; Geais, L.; Astoin, E.; Simondi, M. & Lavaste, F. (2000). The anatomic basis for the concept of lateralized femoral stems: a frontal plane radiographic study of the proximal femur. *The Journal of Arthroplasty*, Vol.15, No.1, (January 2000), pp. 93-101, ISSN 0883-5403

McTighe, T.; Woodgate, I.; Turnbull, A.; Keggi, J.; Kennon, R.; Keppler, L.; Harrison, J.; Brazil, D.; Wu, W. & Cameron, H. U. (2008). A New Approach To Neck Sparing THA Stem. *AAOS Scientific Exhibit*, San Francisco, March 2008

Paliwal, M.; Gordon Allan, D. & Filip, P. (2010). Failure analysis of three uncemented titanium-alloy modular total hip stems. *Engineering Failure Analysis*, Vol.17, No.5, (July 2010), pp. 1230-1238, ISSN 1350-6307

Sharan, D. (1999). The problem of corrosion in orthopaedic implant materials. *Orthopaedic Update (India)*, Vol.9, No.1, (December 1999), pp. 1-5

Shetty, R. (1989). *Use of Dissimilar Metals in Orthopaedic Implants*, Zimmer, Inc., Retrieved from http://www.zimmer.co.nz/web/enUS/pdf/Use_Of_Dissimilar_Metals_in_Orthopaedic_Implants.pdf>

Skendzel, J. G.; Blaha, J. D. & Urquhart, A. G. (2011). Total hip arthroplasty modular neck failure. *The Journal of Arthroplasty*, Vol.26, No.2, (February 2011), pp. 338.e1-338.e4

Toni, A.; Paderni, S.; Sudanese, A.; Guerra, E.; Traina, F.; Antonietti, B. & Giunti, A. (2001). Anatomic cementless total hip arthroplasty with ceramic bearings and modular necks: 3 to 5 years follow-up. *Hip International*, Vol.11, No.1, (2001), pp. 1-17

Traina, F.; De Clerico, M.; Biondi, F.; Pilla, F.; Tassinari, E. & Toni, A. (2009). Sex differences in hip morphology: is stem modularity effective for total hip replacement? *The Journal of Bone and Joint Surgery*, Vol.91, Suppl.6, (November 2009), pp. 121-128

Wilson, D. J.; Dunbar, M.; Amirault, J. & Farhat, Z. (2010). Early failure of a modular femoral neck total hip arthroplasty component: a case report. *The Journal of Bone and Joint Surgery*, Vol.92, No.6, (June 2010), pp. 1514-1517

Wilson, N.; Schneller, E.; Montgomery, K. & Bozic, K. (2008). Hip and knee implants: current trends and policy considerations. *Health Affairs*, Vol.27, No.6, (2008), pp. 1587-1598

Wright, G.; Sporer, S.; Urban, R. & Jacobs, J. (2010). Fracture of a Modular Femoral Neck After Total Hip Arthroplasty. A Case Report. *The Journal of Bone and Joint Surgery*, Vol.92, No.6, (June 2010), pp. 1518–1521

Wright Medical Technology, Inc. (2010). Masters Hip Post Training Document, Amsterdam, July 2010

13

Retrograde Stem Removal Techniques in Revision Hip Surgery

Kálmán Tóth
Department of Orthopaedics, University of Szeged
Hungary

1. Introduction

Total hip replacement has about a 50 year old past. In recent decades the number of revision hip arthroplasties in developed countries reached 15-20% of primary replacements. The average survival for both cemented and uncemented implants is about 94-95% at ten years. At the end of that period they have to be replaced.

Removal of a well cemented femoral stem in revision total hip arthroplasty is a technically demanding procedure, which requires knowledge and proficiency in the usage of a multitude of surgical techniques and instruments. Experiences with traditional cement removing techniques have been published in numerous publications (Dennis et al., 1987; Ferguson, 1988; Laffargue et al., 2000; Lauer et al., 2002; Stühmer, 1987).

Femoral component failure and fracture is a rarely seen complication, which presents as a difficult problem for the surgical team. Because of stress shielding in the proximal femur, osteolysis is often concentrated to the proximal part of the femur, whilst the distal portion of the stem might be stable and well fixed. This eventually leads to failure of the metal and component fracture. Although removing the proximal loose fragment is relatively straightforward, removing the distal tip is difficult, and often only feasible with techniques that result in weakening of the biomechanical properties of the femur, such as distal fenestration i.e. creating a small or larger window (in the lateral cortex or an extended trochanteric osteotomy (Wagner, 1989).

The Authors use a retrograde technique in the clinical setting, in which removal of cement and stem is performed with the use of a retrograde nail passed through the knee. With this technique, removal of loose stems or broken components is both possible – when the case is appropriate for the technique. Thus further compromise can be avoided to the poor bone stock.

2. Surgical technique

The patients were positioned supine on a radio-lucent table. Using a lateral approach, the scar tissue was excised and the hip joint was exposed. After dislocating the prosthesis, the proximal broken piece of the femoral component was easily removed. The end of the distal part became visible at approximately 4 to 6 cm below the lesser trochanter (Fig. 1.).

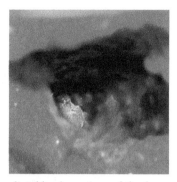

Fig. 1. The proximal end of the distal broken piece of the femoral component - there is no sufficient gap between the broken component and the femur, therefore grasping and pulling it out with a device is not feasible (intraoperative photo).

A 2-3 cm skin incision was required through the centre of the patellar ligament as described by Moed et al. (Moed & Watson, 1995) which is generally performed for osteosynthesis. The optimal entry point for retrograde femoral nailing and defined this spot 12 mm anterior to the femoral origin of the posterior cruciate ligament in sagittal plane and at the centre of the intercondylar sulcus in coronal plane. The intramedullary canal was then opened by the awl.

Under the control of a fluoroscope the 10, 12, 14 mm intramedullary nail is entered into the intramedullary canal. Reaming is not necessary, the tamp that fits best the intramedullary canal is chosen from the series. After entering the rod, it is rotated until the best alignment is obtained to the stem or the cement plug and a stable connection is achieved (Fig. 2.). To avoid deflection or perforation it is particularly important to make sure that the nail is not

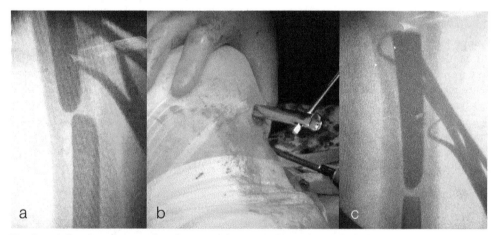

Fig. 2. a: After introducing, the alignment between the nail and the stem is poor, therefore the nail may slip from the tip of the stem causing perforation or fracture (photo taken from the image intensifier). b: Setting the rotation (intraoperative photo). c: After the nail is placed to the tip of the stem the femoral component is removed by gentle hammering (photo taken from the image intensifier).

slipped down from the stem or the distal cement plug. When the required contact between the nail and the distal part of the stem or the cement plug is visualised by the image intensifier, the femoral implant is pushed out in proximal direction by careful hammering.

Following this, the femur was reamed with a cannulated femoral reamer from the proximal end until all the granulation tissue and cement debris was removed. The intramedullary nail was pulled back during reaming without removing it from the distal femur, in order to protect the knee joint from cement particles. After thorough cleaning of the medullary canal the new femoral component was implanted. Using this method, the cortical bone is not weakened and in most cases a normal femoral stem gives sufficient stability for the revision (Fig. 3.).

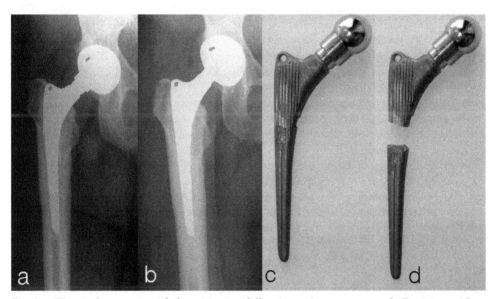

Fig. 3. a: Femoral component failure 14 years following primary surgery. b: Revision with normal femoral component following retrograde removal of broken stem. c and d: Removed, broken component.

The perioperative protocol (thrombopropylaxis, one-shot antibiotic prophylaxis, and applying antibiotic bone cement in case of cemented refixation) does not differ from the routine procedure. Occasional knee swelling occurring in the immediate postoperative period can be treated with local ice packs and applying non-steroidal anti-inflammatory drugs. Physiotherapy and mobilisation does not alter from the routine postoperative protocol.

3. Discussion

When performing revision THR, removal of the distal, often inaccessible cement or a distal fragment of a broken femoral stem is a significant concern (Engh et al., 1999). Whilst intraoperative femoral fracture remains a rare but serious complication during primary

THR, it is a significant problem during revisions (1% of 23,980 primary total hip arthroplasties compared with 7.8% of 6349 revisions in a study by Berry (Berry, 1999)). Subsequent studies have demonstrated similar results (Davis et al., 2003; Egan & Cesare, 1995; Mitchell et al., 2003; Sarvilinna et al., 2004; Taylor et al., 1978).

Farfalli (Farfalli et al., 2007) reported a series of fifty-nine intraoperative fractures that had occurred during revision total hip arthroplasty using impaction bone-grafting. The majority of the fractures (44%) occurred during cement removal.

Various new techniques have been introduced to lower the incidence of perioperative femoral fractures during cement removal, such as ultrasound (Caillouette et al., 1991; Honnart, 1996; Klapper et al., 1992; Schwaller & Elke, 2001), extra-corporal lithotripsy (Braun et al., 1992; Schmidt et al., 1998; Schreurs et al., 1991; Stranne et al., 1992; Weinstein et al., 1988), segmental cement extraction (Chin et al., 1991; Ekelund, 1992; Jingushi et al., 2000; Schurman & Maloney, 1992), application of high-energy shock waves (May et al., 1990), using a ballistically driven chiselling system (Porsch & Schmidt, 2001), or an acoustic emission-controlled milling device (Schmidt & Nordmann, 1994) or even lasers (Sherk et al., 1995). Most of these techniques had not reached widespread usage, and some authors have reported complications (Gardiner et al., 1993).

There have been three clinical studies and one experimental work published about retrograde stem removal (Piatek et al., 2007; Szendroi et al., 2010; Toth et al., 2010; Tóth et al., 2011). Tóth (Toth et al., 2010) and Szendrői (Szendroi et al., 2010) reports successful, uncomplicated application of retrograde removal technique with intact stems and distal fractured components in treatment of elective hip arthroplasty revisions, while Piatek (Piatek et al., 2007) used the technique successfully in case of periprotetic fractures.

The cadaver study compares the biomechanical effects of three different cement removing techniques, the distal fenestration (DF), the transfemoral approach (TFA) and the retrograde stem removal technique (RSR) using an experimental setup (Tóth et al., 2011). 23 paired femora were recovered from similarly aged human cadavers and were frozen. These were later subdivided into 3 groups to provide specimens of similar age and bone quality in each group (DF, TFA, RSR).

The results of the intragroup (comparison between treated and control specimens from the same cadavers from the same groups) analysis were the following: In the TFA group, the force required till fracture was significantly less than in controls (p=0.0096). Similar results were found in the DF group (p=0.068). There was no difference in the RSR group (p=0.988).

Intergroup analysis showed the following:

Femurs in the DF group required significantly less force to fracture than specimens in the RSR (p=0.043), whilst there was no difference in there respective controls (p=0.831).

Femurs in the TFA group required highly significantly less force to fracture than specimens in the RSR group (p=0.0001), whilst there was no difference in there respective controls (p=0.178).

That is, the cadaveric study supports the clinical experience that windowing the proximal femur, significantly decreases resistance against compression and rotational forces.

The various windowing techniques described in the literature (Arif et al., 2004; Buehler & Walker, 1998; Cameron, 1990; Hackenbroch, 1979; Kerry et al., 1999; Klein & Rubash, 1993; Moreland et al., 1986; Nelson & Barnes, 1990; Nelson & Weber, 1980; Savvidis & Löer, 1989;

Shepherd & Turnbull, 1989; Stranne et al., 1992; Tyer et al., 1987; Weber, 1981; Witt & Hackenbroch, 1976), and their modifications (Arif et al., 2004; Nelson & Barnes, 1990; Zweymüller et al., 2005) and the new instruments developed for these techniques (Brinckmann & Horst, 1985), all serve one purpose, to decrease the often inevitable weakening of the proximal femoral bone stock, preserving as much intact bone as possible. Although the more conservative windowing techniques tend to preserve more proximal bone, they still inevitably lead to decreased resistance against fracture.

The studies performed by Dennis et al. (Dennis et al., 1987) on cadaveric femora, showed that when femurs without intramedullary support are stressed to failure, fractures occur through the cortical holes 90% of the time, therefore they suggested that long revision femoral stems should be used to bypass the window by at least 2 to 2.5 times the cortical diameter measured at the fenestration level (Fig. 4/b). This has been generally accepted and is widely used in orthopaedic practice (Kerry et al., 1999; Klein & Rubash, 1993; Lotke et al., 1986; Moreland et al., 1986; Nelson & Barnes, 1990; Nelson & Weber, 1980; Savvidis & Löer, 1989; Shepherd & Turbull, 1989; Tyer et al., 1987).

The disadvantage of using a long stem with proximal opening of the femur instead of the RSR technique and a short stem (Fig. 3a, 3b.), is that long revision stems are more expensive, the necessary exposure requires a longer incision (Fig. 4c), with more soft tissue stripping, surgery is often much longer, blood loss can be extensive, and the local and general complication rate is higher.

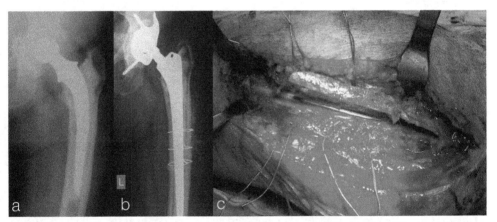

Fig. 4. a: Femoral component failure and acetabular component loosening 17 years following primary surgery. b: Distal fragment of cement and stem are removed through bone window, followed by wire refixation of the window. The long revision femoral stem distally overreaches the window by the length of 2.5 times. c: Major surgical wound with extended osteotomy (intraoperative photo).

The RSR technique cannot always be used, and is absolutely contraindicated in the case of septic loosening or if the knee or the distal femur is affected by primary or metastatic tumours. Large distal cement plugs or the presence of oblique cement at the end of the stem are relative contraindications, because these can force the nail used for removal towards the cortical bone, which can lead to unwanted perforation or even periprosthetic fracture.

In the clinical setting depending on the quality of the proximal femoral bone, both a short a long femoral stem can be used for the revision surgery after RSR. As the cortex is not violated during component removal, a short primary stem (cemented or uncemented) is a valid option and is our preference, if the cortices are not very thin, and at least some peripheral cancellous bone is present, for cement penetration. We like to reserve long stems as a final resort, to allow a possible future revision.

4. Conclusion

Our cadaver experiments clearly confirm the clinical experience, that the window technique significantly weakens resistance of femur against rotation under compression forces. In contrast, with the retrograde cement removal technique this weakening does not occur.

Our experience with retrograde cement removal in elective revisions and periprosthetic fractures shows that - taking into consideration indications and contraindications- retrograde prosthesis removal technique is a viable alternative solution in case of intact as well as failed femoral components. It is associated with less intraoperative complications and faster, safer recovery compared to traditional techniques.

However, longer follow-up time is required to confirm the durability of the observed clinical outcomes.

5. References

Arif, M., Sivananthan, S., & Choon, DS. (2004). Revision of total hip arthroplasty using an anterior cortical window, extensive strut allografts, and an impaction graft: follow-up study. *J Orthop Surg (Hong Kong)*, Vol. 12, No. 1, (June, 2004), pp. 25-30, ISSN 1022-5536

Berry, DJ. (1999). Epidemiology: hip and knee. *Orthop Clin North Am*, Vol. 30, No. 2, (April, 1999), pp. 183-190, ISSN 0030-5898

Braun, W., Claes, L., Ruter, A., & Paschke, D. (1992). Effect of shock waves on the strength of connection between bone and polymethylmethacrylate. An in vitro study of human femur segments. *Z Orthop Ihre Grenzgeb*, Vol. 130, No. 3, (May-June, 1992), pp. 236-243, ISSN 0044-3220

Brinckmann, P., & Horst, M. (1985). New instruments for the removal of an artificial hip joint from the shaft. *Z Orthop Ihre Grenzgeb*, Vol. 123, No. 1, (January-February, 1985), pp. 113-114, ISSN 0044-3220

Buehler, KO., & Walker, RH. (1998). Polymethylmethacrylate removal from the femur using a crescentic window technique. *Orthopedics*, Vol. 21, No. 6, (June, 1998), pp. 697-700, ISSN 0147-7447

Caillouette, JT., Gorab, RS., Klapper, RC., & Anzel, SH. (1991). Revision arthroplasty facilitated by ultrasonic tool cement removal. Part II: histologic analysis of endosteal bone after cement removal. *Orthop Rev*, Vol. 20, No. 5, (May, 1991), pp. 435-440, ISSN 0094-6591

Cameron, HU. (1990). Tips of the trade #29. Femoral windows for easy cement removal in hip revision surgery. *Orthop Rev*, Vol. 19, No. 10, (October, 1990), pp. 909-910, 912 ISSN 0094-6591

Chin, AK., Moll, FH., McColl, MB., Hoffman, KJ., & Wuh, HC. (1991). An improved technique for cement extraction in revision total hip arthroplasty. *Contemp Orthop*, Vol. 22, No. 3, (March, 1991), pp. 255-264, ISSN 0194-8458

Davis, CM., 3rd, Berry, DJ., & Harmsen, WS. (2003). Cemented revision of failed uncemented femoral components of total hip arthroplasty. *J Bone Joint Surg Am*, Vol. 85-A, No. 7, (July, 2003), pp.1264-1269, ISSN 0021-9355

Dennis, DA., Dingman, CA., Meglan, DA., O'Leary, JF., Mallory, TH., & Berme, N. (1987). Femoral cement removal in revision total hip arthroplasty. A biomechanical analysis. *Clin Orthop Relat Res*, Vol. 220, No. 7, (July, 1987), pp. 142-147, ISSN 0009-921X

Egan, KJ., & Di Cesare, PE. (1995). Intraoperative complications of revision hip arthroplasty using a fully porous-coated straight cobalt-chrome femoral stem. *J Arthroplasty*, Vol. 10, Suppl. (November, 1995), pp. 45-51, ISSN 0883-5403

Ekelund, AL. (1992). Cement removal in revision hip arthroplasty. Experience with bone cement added to the cavity in 20 cases. *Acta Orthop Scand*, Vol. 63, No. 5, (October, 1992), pp. 549-551, ISSN 0001-6470

Engh, CA., McAuley, JP., & Engh, C. (1999). Surgical approaches for revision total hip replacement surgery: the anterior trochanteric slide and the extended conventional osteotomy. *Instr Course Lect*, Vol. 48, (1999), pp. 3-8, ISSN 0065-6895

Farfalli, GL., Buttaro, MA., & Piccaluga, F. (2007). Femoral fractures in revision hip surgeries with impacted bone allograft. *Clin Orthop Relat Res*, Vol. 462, No. 9, (September, 2007), pp. 130-136, ISSN 0009-921X

Ferguson, GM. (1988). Femoral cement removal in revision total hip arthroplasty: a biomechanical analysis. *Clin Orthop Relat Res*, Vol. 234, No. 8, (September, 1998), pp. 307-308, ISSN 0009-921X

Gardiner, R., Hozack, WJ., Nelson, C., & Keating, EM. (1993). Revision total hip arthroplasty using ultrasonically driven tools. A clinical evaluation *J Arthroplasty*, Vol. 8, No. 5, (October, 1993), pp. 517-521, ISSN 0883-5403

Hackenbroch, Jr. MH. (1979). Possibilities and limitations of exchange of hip and knee joint prostheses. *Z Orthop Ihre Grenzgeb*, Vol. 117, No. 4, (August, 1979), pp. 457-460, ISSN 0044-3220

Honnart, F. (1996). Use of ultrasound for the removal of cement in hip prosthesis reoperations. *Rev Chir Orthop Reparatrice Appar Mot*, Vol. 82, No. 2, (1996), pp. 171-174, ISSN 0035-1040

Jingushi, S., Noguchi, Y., Shuto, T., Nakashima, T., & Iwamoto Y. (2000). A device for removal of femoral distal cement plug during hip revision arthroplasty: a high-powered drill equipped with a centralizer. *J Arthroplasty*, Vol. 15, No. 2, (February, 2000), pp. 231-233, ISSN 0883-5403

Kerry, RM., Masri, BA., Garbuz, DS., & Duncan, CP. (1999). The vascularized scaphoid window for access to the femoral canal in revision total hip arthroplasty. *Instr Course Lect*, Vol. 48, (1999), pp. 9-11, ISSN 0065-6895

Klapper, RC., Caillouette, JT., Callaghan, JJ., & Hozack, WJ. (1992). Ultrasonic technology in revision joint arthroplasty. *Clin Orthop*, Vol. 285, No. 12, (December, 1992), pp. 147-154, ISSN 0009-921X

Klein, AH., & Rubash, HE. (1993). Femoral windows in revision total hip arthroplasty. *Clin Orthop Relat Res*, Vol. 291, No. 6, (June, 1993), pp. 164-170, ISSN 0009-921X

Laffargue, P., De Lestang, M., Bonnomet, F., Dupart, L., & Havet, E. (2000). Techniques of component and cement removal: osseous pitfalls and approaches. *Rev Chir Orthop Reparatrice Appar Mot*, Vol. 86, No. 9, Suppl. (September, 2000), pp. 51-54, ISSN 0035-1040

Lauer, W., Neuss, M., Wirtz, DC., & Radermacher, K. (2002). Technical principles for removal of femoral bone cements in hip prosthesis implant revision. *Biomed Tech (Berl)*, Vol. 47, Suppl 1 Pt, (2002), pp. 47-48, ISSN 0013-5585

Lotke, PA., Wong, RY., & Ecker, ML. (1986). Stress fracture as a cause of chronic pain following revision total hip arthroplasty. Report of two cases. Clin Orthop Relat Res, Vol. 206, (May, 1986) pp. 147-150, ISSN 0009-921X

May, TC., Krause, WR., Preslar, AJ., Smith, MJ., Beaudoin, AJ., & Cardea, JA. (1990). Use of high-energy shock waves for bone cement removal. *J Arthroplasty*, Vol. 5, No. 1, (March, 1990), pp. 19-27, ISSN 0883-5403

Mitchell, PA., Greidanus, NV., Masri, BA., Garbuz, DS., & Duncan, CP. (2003). The prevention of periprosthetic fractures of the femur during and after total hip arthroplasty. *Instr Course Lect*, Vol. 52, (2003), pp. 301-308, ISSN 0065-6895

Moed, BR., & Watson JT. (1995). Retrograde intramedullary nailing, without reaming, of fractures of the femoral shaft in multiply injure patient. *J. Bone Joint Surg. Am*, Vol. 75, No.10, (October, 1995), pp. 1520-1527, ISSN 0021-9355

Moreland, JR., Marder, R., & Anspach, WE Jr. (1986). The window technique for the removal of broken femoral stems in total hip replacement. *Clin Orthop Relat Res*, Vol.212, (November, 1986), pp. 245-249, ISSN 0009-921X

Nelson, CL., & Weber, MJ. (1981). Technique of windowing the femoral shaft for removal of bone cement. *Clin Orthop Relat Res*, Vol. 154, (January-February, 1981), pp. 336-337 ISSN 0009-921X

Nelson, CL., & Barnes, CL. (1990). Removal of bone cement from the femoral shaft using a femoral windowing device. J Arthroplasty, Vol. 5, No. 1, (March, 1990), pp. 67-69, ISSN 0883-5403

Piatek, S., Westphal, T., Holmenschlager, F., Becker, R, & Winckler, S. (2007). Retrograde cement removal in periprosthetic fractures following hip arthroplasty. *Arch Orthop Trauma Surg*, Vol. 127, No. 7, (September, 2007), pp. 581-585, ISSN 0936-8051

Porsch, M., & Schmidt, J. (2001). Cement removal with an endoscopically controlled ballistically driven chiselling system. A new device for cement removal and preliminary clinical results. *Arch Orthop Trauma Surg*, Vol. 121, No. 5, (May, 2001), pp. 274–277, ISSN:0936-8051

Sarvilinna, R., Huhtala, HS., Sovelius, RT., Halonen, PJ., Nevalainen, JK., & Pajam"aki, KJ. (2004). Factors predisposing to periprosthetic fracture after hip arthroplasty: a case (n = 31)-control study. Acta Orthop Scand, Vol. 75 No. 1, (February, 2004), pp. 16-20, ISSN 0001-6470

Savvidis, E., & Löer, F. (1989). Surgical technique for femur shaft fenestration in revisional surgery following total hip replacements – a comparative experimental study. *Z Orthop Ihre Grenzgeb*, Vol. 127, No. 2, (1989), pp. 228-236, ISSN 0044-3220

Schreurs, BW., Bierkens, AF., Huiskes, R., Hendrikx, AJ., & Slooff, TJ. (1991). The effect of the extracorporeal shock wave lithotriptor on bone cement. *J Biomed Mater Res*, Vol. 25, No. 2, (February, 1991), pp. 157–164, ISSN 0021-9304

Schmidt, J., & Nordmann, K. (1994). Removal of bone cement from the femoral canal using an acoustic emission-controlled milling device. *Med Biol Eng Comput*, Vol. 32, No. 3, (May, 1994), pp. 258-260, ISSN 0140-0118

Schmidt, J., Porsch, M., Hackenbroch, MH., Koebke, J., & Brimmers, P. (1998). ModiWed intracorporeal lithotripsy for cement removal in hip prosthesis exchange operations–experimental principles. *Z Orthop Ihre Grenzgeb*, Vol. 136, No. 1, (January-February, 1998), pp. 44-49, ISSN 0044-3220

Schurman, DJ., & Maloney, WJ. (1992). Segmental cement extraction at revision total hip arthroplasty. *Clin Orthop*, Vol. 285, (December, 1992), pp. 158-163, ISSN:0009-921X

Schwaller, CA., & Elke, R. (2001). Cement removal with ultrasound in revision or total hip prosthesis. *Orthopade*, Vol. 30, No. 5, (May, 2001), pp. 310-316, ISSN:0085-4530

Shepherd, BD., & Turnbull, A. (1989). The fate of femoral windows in revision joint arthroplasty. *J Bone Joint Surg Am*, Vol. 71, No. 5, (June, 1989), pp. 716-718, ISSN 0021-9355

Sherk, HH., Lane, G., Rhodes, A., & Black, J. (1995). Carbon dioxide laser removal of polymethylmethacrylate. *Clin Orthop, Vol. 310, (January, 1995), pp.* 67-71, ISSN 0009-921X

Stranne, SK., Callaghan, JJ., Fyda, TM., Fulghum, CS., Glisson, RR., Weinerth, JL., & Seaber, AV. (1992). The effect of extracorporeal shock wave lithotripsy on the prosthesis interface in cementless arthroplasty. Evaluation in a rabbit model. *J Arthroplasty*, Vol. 7, No. 2, (June, 1992), pp. 173-179, ISSN 0883-5403

Stühmer, K. (1987). Zur Technik der Zemententfernung bei Austauschoperationen von Gelenkendoprothesen. *Aktuel Probl Chir Orthop*, Vol. 31, (1987), pp. 342-346, ISSN 0378-8504

Szendrői, M., Tóth, K., Kiss, J., Antal, I., & Skaliczki G. (2010). Retrograde genocephalic removal of fractured or immovable femoral stems in revision hip surgery. *Hip Int.* Vol. 20, No. 1, (January-March, 2010), pp. 34-37, ISSN 1120-7000

Taylor, MM., Meyers, MH., & Harvey, JP Jr. (1978). Intraoperative femur fractures during total hip replacement. *Clin Orthop Relat Res*, Vol. 137, (November-December, 1978), pp. 96-103, ISSN 0009-921X

Toth, K., Sisak, K., Nagy, J., Mano, S., & Csernatony, Z. (2010). Retrograde stem removal in revision hip surgery: removing a loose or broken femoral component with a retrograde nail. *Archives of Orthopaedic and Trauma Surgery*, Vol. 130, No. 7, (July, 2010), pp. 813-818, ISSN 0936-8051

Tóth, K., Sisák, K., Wellinger, K., Manó, S., Horváth, G., Szendrői, M., & Csernátony, Z. (2011). Biomechanical comparison of three cemented stem removal techniques in revision hip surgery. *Arch Orthop Trauma Surg.* Vol. 131, No. 7, (July, 2011), pp. 1007-1012, ISSN 0936-8051

Tyer, HD., Huckstep, RL., & Stalley, PD. (1987). Intraluminal allograft restoration of the upper femur in failed total hip arthroplasty. *Clin Orthop Relat Res*, Vol. 224, (November, 1987), pp. 26-32, ISSN 0009-921X

Wagner, H. (1989). A revision prosthesis for the hip joint. *Orthopade*, Vol. 18, No. 5, (September, 1989), pp. 438-453, ISSN 0085-4530

Weber, BG. (1981). Total hip replacement revision surgery: Surgical technique and experience. In: *Hip*, E.A. Salvati, (Ed.), 3-14, Proceedings of the 9th Open Scientific Meeting of the Hip Society, ISBN 0095-7216, St. Louis, Mosby, USA

Weinstein, JN., Oster, DM., Park, JB., Park, SH., & Loening, S. (1988). The effect of the extracorporeal shock wave lithotriptor on the bone-cement interface in dogs. *Clin Orthop*, Vol. 235, (October, 1988), pp. 261–267, ISSN 0009-921X

Witt, AN., & Hackenbroch, MH. (1976). Therapeutic approaches to implant loosening in total hip arthroplasty. *Z Orthop Ihre Grenzgeb*, Vol. 114, No. 3, (June, 1976), pp. 330-341, ISSN 0044-3220

Zweymüller, KA., Steindl, M., & Melmer, T. (2005). Anterior windowing of the femur diaphysis for cement removal in revision surgery. *Clin Orthop Relat Res*, Vol. 441, (December, 2005), pp. 227-336, ISSN 0009-921X

Permissions

The contributors of this book come from diverse backgrounds, making this book a truly international effort. This book will bring forth new frontiers with its revolutionizing research information and detailed analysis of the nascent developments around the world.

We would like to thank Dr. Samo K. Fokter, MD, for lending his expertise to make the book truly unique. He has played a crucial role in the development of this book. Without his invaluable contribution this book wouldn't have been possible. He has made vital efforts to compile up to date information on the varied aspects of this subject to make this book a valuable addition to the collection of many professionals and students.

This book was conceptualized with the vision of imparting up-to-date information and advanced data in this field. To ensure the same, a matchless editorial board was set up. Every individual on the board went through rigorous rounds of assessment to prove their worth. After which they invested a large part of their time researching and compiling the most relevant data for our readers. Conferences and sessions were held from time to time between the editorial board and the contributing authors to present the data in the most comprehensible form. The editorial team has worked tirelessly to provide valuable and valid information to help people across the globe.

Every chapter published in this book has been scrutinized by our experts. Their significance has been extensively debated. The topics covered herein carry significant findings which will fuel the growth of the discipline. They may even be implemented as practical applications or may be referred to as a beginning point for another development. Chapters in this book were first published by InTech; hereby published with permission under the Creative Commons Attribution License or equivalent.

The editorial board has been involved in producing this book since its inception. They have spent rigorous hours researching and exploring the diverse topics which have resulted in the successful publishing of this book. They have passed on their knowledge of decades through this book. To expedite this challenging task, the publisher supported the team at every step. A small team of assistant editors was also appointed to further simplify the editing procedure and attain best results for the readers.

Our editorial team has been hand-picked from every corner of the world. Their multi-ethnicity adds dynamic inputs to the discussions which result in innovative outcomes. These outcomes are then further discussed with the researchers and contributors who give their valuable feedback and opinion regarding the same. The feedback is then collaborated with the researches and they are edited in a comprehensive manner to aid the understanding of the subject.

Apart from the editorial board, the designing team has also invested a significant amount of their time in understanding the subject and creating the most relevant covers. They scrutinized every image to scout for the most suitable representation of the subject and create an appropriate cover for the book.

The publishing team has been involved in this book since its early stages. They were actively engaged in every process, be it collecting the data, connecting with the contributors or procuring relevant information. The team has been an ardent support to the editorial, designing and production team. Their endless efforts to recruit the best for this project, has resulted in the accomplishment of this book. They are a veteran in the field of academics and their pool of knowledge is as vast as their experience in printing. Their expertise and guidance has proved useful at every step. Their uncompromising quality standards have made this book an exceptional effort. Their encouragement from time to time has been an inspiration for everyone.

The publisher and the editorial board hope that this book will prove to be a valuable piece of knowledge for researchers, students, practitioners and scholars across the globe.

List of Contributors

N. A. Sandiford and U. Alao
Specialist Registrar, Kent and Sussex Hospital, Mount Ephraim, Tunbridge Wells, Kent, United Kingdom

J. A. Skinner
Consultant Orthopaedic surgeon Royal National Orthopaedic, Hospital Brockley Hill, Stanmore, United Kingdom

S. R. Samsani
Consultant Orthopaedic surgeon, Medway Maritime Hospital, Windmill Road, Gillingham, Kent, United Kingdom

Antonio Silvestre, Fernando Almeida, Pablo Renovell, Raúl López, Laura Pino and Luis Puertes
School of Medicine Valencia/Hospital Clínico Valencia, Spain

Ahmed Alghamdi and Martin Lavigne
Université de Montréal, Canada

Samo K. Fokter
Celje General and Teaching Hospital, Slovenia

Nina Fokter
Maribor University Clinical Centre, Slovenia

Mel S. Lee
College of Medicine, Chang Gung University, Department of Orthopedic Surgery, Chang Gung Memorial Hospital at Linkou, Taiwan

Andrej Strahovnik and Samo K. Fokter
General and Teaching Hospital Celje, Slovenia

Tosan Okoro and Peter Maddison
Bangor University, United Kingdom
Ysbyty Gwynedd, Betsi Cadwaladr,University Health Board, Bangor, United Kingdom

John G. Andrew
Ysbyty Gwynedd, Betsi Cadwaladr, University Health Board, Bangor, United Kingdom

Andrew Lemmey
Bangor University, United Kingdom

Magdalena Wilk-Frańczuk
Frycz-Modrzewski Cracow University, Cracow Rehabilitation Center, Scanmed St. Rafael Hospital, Cracow, Poland

Hiran Amarasekera
Orthopaedic Research Fellow/PhD Student, Warwick Orthopaedics, University of Warwick Medical School, United Kingdom

Damian Griffin
Professor of Trauma and Orthopaedics, Warwick Orthopaedics, University of Warwick Medical School, United Kingdom

Nevzat Selim Gokay and Alper Gokce
Namik Kemal University School of Medicine, Department of Orthopaedics and Traumatology, Tekirdag, Turkey

Bulent Alp and Fahri Erdogan
Istanbul University, Cerrahpasa School of Medicine, Department of Orthopaedics and Traumatology, Istanbul, Turkey

Zoran Bascarevic and Zoran Vukasinovic
Faculty of Medicine, University of Belgrade, Belgrade, Serbia
Institute of Orthopaedic Surgery „Banjica", Belgrade, Serbia

Violeta Bascarevic
Institute of Orthopaedic Surgery „Banjica", Belgrade, Serbia

Vladimir Bascarevic
Faculty of Medicine, University of Belgrade, Belgrade, Serbia
Institute of Neurosurgery, Clinical Center of Serbia, Belgrade, Serbia

Igor Vučajnk and Samo K. Fokter
Celje General and Teaching Hospital, Slovenia

Kálmán Tóth
Department of Orthopaedics, University of Szeged, Hungary